Praise for *Sex, Health, and Consciousness*

"In *Sex, Health, and Consciousness*, Liz Goldwyn gives us an inspiring vision of a world where our sacred sexuality isn't something to hide—but something to cherish and nurture. Liz artfully guides all of us toward this new normal, with tools and skill-building that unleash healthy pleasure and provide us with a more expansive definition of full-body health. Read this book, and watch your sexuality flourish."

EMILY MORSE

doctor of human sexuality, CEO & founder of Sex with Emily

"*Sex, Health, and Consciousness* offers an approachable, welcoming path to opening your mind to new ways of thinking around sexuality, allowing the reader to discover for themselves what is possible. Liz is a nurturing companion for the ride, sharing her hard-won wisdom, vulnerability, and often hilarious experiences along the way."

MARISA TOMEI

Academy Award-winning actress, activist

"In *Sex, Health, and Consciousness*, Liz introduces a new, expanded approach to sexual liberation that urges the reader to explore sexuality through a holistic, fully embodied state of emotional, physical, and spiritual well-being."

SOPHIA AMORUSO

New York Times bestselling author of *#Girlboss*

"With humor and unflinching honesty about her own struggles and awakenings, Liz brings down to earth topics most of us are uncomfortable asking about. *Sex, Health, and Consciousness* is full of helpful information and practical advice, discussing the complexities of human sexuality with compassion, clarity, and, most importantly, an absence of shame."

TONY GOLDWYN

actor, director, producer

"Whether recounting stories from surfer buddies, her dying father, or burlesque queens of the past, Liz Goldwyn imparts the wisdom she has learned about sex from her extensive research and life experiences to her reader in the most inspired yet relatable way possible. *Sex, Health, and Consciousness* is a collection of lived experiences, not just of the author but of the many sexperts she's had the privilege of knowing and interviewing over the years. The book ties together history, myth, religion and spirituality, comedy, porn, pop culture, technology, and the environment to allow its reader to ascend to a greater understanding of the power sex has in each of our lives. One walks away from this book with a better understanding about how to appreciate the changes our bodies and mind go through over time and how sex and sexuality are key ingredients to a happier and healthier existence."

JOSHUA GONZALEZ, MD

board-certified urologist, specialist in sexual medicine

"Liz Goldwyn has done it again! *Sex, Health, and Consciousness* is sure to reinvent the way you think about intimacy, relationships, and yourself."

NATASHA LYONNE

actress, director, writer, producer

SEX · HEALTH & CONSCIOUSNESS

ALSO BY LIZ GOLDWYN

Pretty Things: The Last Generation of American Burlesque Queens

Sporting Guide: Los Angeles, 1897

SEX · HEALTH & CONSCIOUSNESS

MEDITATE MASTURBATE MANIFEST · REPARENT REPROGRAM · REJOICE IN YOUR · FREE YOUR MIND AND YOUR ASS WILL FOLLOW · TRANSFORM · EVOLVE · SELF LOVE · SELF ESTEEM · TRANSCEND · EXPAND YOUR PLEASURE · YOUR ORGASM

LIZ GOLDWYN

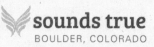

sounds true

BOULDER, COLORADO

Sounds True is a trademark of Sounds True, Inc.

Published 2022

Cover design by Jennifer Miles
Book design by Linsey Dodaro

Printed in the United States of America

BK06453

Library of Congress Cataloging-in-Publication Data
Names: Goldwyn, Liz, author.
Title: Sex, health, and consciousness : how to reclaim your pleasure
    potential / by Liz Goldwyn.
Description: Boulder, CO : Sounds True, 2022. | Includes bibliographical
    references.
Identifiers: LCCN 2022007407 (print) | LCCN 2022007408 (ebook) |
    ISBN 9781683649458 (trade paperback) | ISBN 9781683649465 (ebook)
Subjects: LCSH: Sex. | Sex instruction. | Sexual health. | Sexual
    excitement.
Classification: LCC HQ21 .G626 2022 (print) | LCC HQ21 (ebook) |
    DDC 613.9/6--dc23/eng/20220520
LC record available at https://lccn.loc.gov/2022007407
LC ebook record available at https://lccn.loc.gov/2022007408

FSC
www.fsc.org
MIX
Paper | Supporting
responsible forestry
FSC® C103098

10 9 8 7 6 5 4 3 2 1

With love and gratitude for all past, present, and
future versions of me, you, and us.

CONTENTS

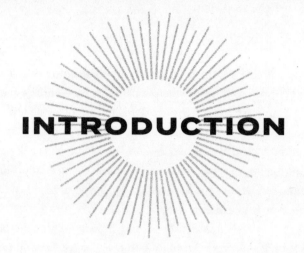

INTRODUCTION

What do you think of when you read the words *sex, health, and consciousness*? Do those seem like three entirely different subjects? If you bought this book in a store or online, did you find it in the self-help/spirituality section, or in wellness, or in sexuality? Have you, like me, ever wondered why these categories are separated from one another? Collectively, we tend to silo our sexuality away from our mind, body, and spirit instead of integrating it. This strikes me as counterintuitive, especially as sex (and love) drives almost every aspect of human existence.

I believe that, as a culture, we need to radically redefine how we think and talk about sex. We need to take an honest look at how often we compartmentalize our sexuality and how disconnected we are from the primal energy (or life force) that our sexuality, and the act of sex itself, holds. Even thinking of sex as an activity that requires another person or must result in an orgasm needs to be questioned.

Sex can be a verb; a noun; a state of mind; an energy; a feeling; a source of power for some, of trauma for others; it can serve as a function of procreation, lust, even transcendence. Can we agree that whatever our current viewpoint, sex is a powerful act, action, or experience? *Health* is an easier word for which to land on a commonly accepted meaning: the condition of being well. What steps do we take to make ourselves healthy? Is it being mindful of the food we eat and of how much exercise and sleep we get? What about our bodily functions, genitalia, orgasms, masturbation, intimacy, and communication with sexual partners? The kind of content we consume and the sex we have? Where does our relationship with technology, pornography, dating, and love fit in? I believe all these parts of being a human in the twenty-first century affect our state of health. Consciousness is the area where most of us have entirely individual ideologies. In the simplest terms, *consciousness* is a state of being awake. For you, this could mean trying to be in the present moment and truly aware of your body, surroundings, and the people around you. Others may think of meditation, yoga, spirituality, or religion. Or maybe you have no relationship to any of the aforementioned terms. This is okay. For our purposes together, let's think of consciousness as heightened awareness.

A deep dive into the intersection of and holistic alignment between sex, health, and consciousness is what follows in these pages. I see our culture's current take on sexuality as kind of like using a twelve-color Crayola box to draw with. A ROYGBIV (red orange yellow green blue indigo violet) rainbow is great, don't get me wrong, but what if colors are missing that could help us create a masterpiece? One that would blow every piece of art we've ever seen out of the water? This book is designed to help you access the latent Michelangelo lurking inside each of you.

To help on this journey, within these pages you will find homework, suggested practices to incorporate into your daily/weekly/monthly routine. You can integrate existing religious or spiritual beliefs into the framework I am laying out, and if you identify as atheist, you are welcome, too! All practices are in invitation, whatever your previous relationship to sex, health, and consciousness—even if you've no prior connection to these topics at all. I encourage you to make the exercises I offer here your own. Only you know best how to move, honor, and pleasure your body and soul.

What makes me the right person to be your guide on this trip?

Let me take you back . . .

I was an endlessly curious kid with an insatiable desire for more knowledge than was deemed age appropriate. I was especially fascinated by this mysterious word, *sex*, that grown-ups spoke of in hushed tones. I recognized from a very early age how much this word drove adult behavior. But no one would or could explain to me what exactly it meant and why everyone was obsessed by and secretive (ashamed) about it.

When I was eleven, I started borrowing my father's *Playboy* magazines, prompted by the appearance of my then idol, Madonna, on the cover. It was our Sunday ritual to go for breakfast at the coffee shop at the Beverly Hills Hotel. Afterward, I would wait for Dad while he got his nails trimmed at the barber salon next door. I got caught lifting the Madonna cover from the salon while he was at his weekly grooming appointment. His manicurist, who was in her late seventies, reprimanded me for looking at photos of naked ladies. I didn't see what was wrong with studying body parts that I'd soon develop myself. How was I supposed to understand anything if grown-ups were keeping me from it?

I soon figured out where my dad stashed his porn mags at home and orchestrated a playdate with the cutest boy in my class to look at *Playboy* together. I took him to my secret hiding place in our backyard, tucked away from prying eyes, and pulled out a centerfold. He freaked out, and I put the magazine away, embarrassed. Later, we went out for ice cream and ran into two other boys from our class. They made fun of us for being on a "date" and asked me if I'd gotten my "pee-red" yet. They were quite proud of their taunts, having just learned what menstruation was a few weeks earlier during the one day of sex education we had in middle school (clearly, an unsuccessful academic exercise). The closest I got to having real sex ed in school was a human development course in seventh grade. Our teacher, a sex-positive hippie, instructed us all to go home and examine our vaginas using hand mirrors.

If I had a specific question about sexuality, my parents did their best to answer me in a way that provided cultural and political context. I recall asking my mother what a "sex change" (now called "gender transitioning")[1] was when I was around nine. She told me about the tennis player Renée Richards, who had transitioned from male to female and became a transgender activist after she fought to compete in the 1976 US Open, paving the way for a landmark New York Supreme Court ruling in her favor. My mother was on the board of Planned Parenthood and active in supporting women's reproductive rights. Yet she and my father—as liberated as they might have thought they were—never sat me down to have a one-on-one sex talk that covered more intimate questions, like "When should I lose my virginity? Would it hurt?" "How would I know if I was in love? Would that hurt, too?" "Was it normal to masturbate? Was there a right way to do it?"

---

1   This term refers to those whose medically assessed sex does not align with their self assessed gender identity and/or sex. These individuals may or may not opt to explore a range of medical options that affirm their self-assessed gender and/or sex (chiefly hormone therapies and gender-affirmation surgeries). Emerging conversations within the trans community consider trans identity less through an event-based lens ("before transition" versus "after transition," "pre-op" versus "post-op") and more through a journey-based lens ("transitioning"), allowing endless personal locations on a trans continuum of identity, experience, and practice.

My first real job was as a paid intern for Planned Parenthood. I was thirteen. Although most of my friends were already losing their virginity, I hadn't even given a blow job, much less "gone all the way." Yet there I was, working in the office at the Santa Monica clinic, in the thick of STI[2] testing with antiabortionists picketing outside—plunged into the deep end of my professional sex education. I played online solitaire while fielding the phones, often antiabortion callers threatening the safety of the clinic and our staff with bomb threats.

Note: as this book goes to print, Roe vs. Wade, the landmark 1973 Supreme Court case that granted Americans the right to a legal abortion has just been overturned. Growing up with a mother who was Education Chairman on the Board of Planned Parenthood-Los Angeles, I don't remember a time where I was not aware of the dark and bloody history of abortion pre Roe vs. Wade. My mother took me to my first Planned Parenthood clinic to help women enter safely amongst the protesters outside when I was around 9 years old. I would overhear her conversations about wire hangers being used by desperate women performing at-home abortions; about the high mortality rates when it was criminalized; about the marches and sweat and tears of her generation as they fought for our right to choose. I understood what it took (and how many women's lives were lost along the way with often dangerous illegal abortions) to win the battle for freedom over our bodies. I never thought I would be mourning this very basic human right being taken away while completing a book whose impetus began when I first started working at a Planned Parenthood clinic all those years ago. As I send these pages to my publisher, we face more threats to our sexual and gender freedom—from expected restrictions on birth control; assisted reproductive technology like IVF and egg freezing; the right to sexual privacy, gay marriage, and more. I shudder to think where we will be by the time you are holding this book in your hands. As angry and heartbroken and tired as I feel in this moment, I will never stop fighting for these rights. I will never stop believing that the more information and education we have around these topics, the more we progress and expand as human beings and as a culture.

At Planned Parenthood, I was in the position of advising other kids about subjects I was in the process of learning about. In the media library of the clinic, it

---

2   This acronym stands for "sexually transmitted infections," or infections that have been spread through sexual contact, typically vaginal, anal, and/or oral. These can include (but are not limited to) chlamydia, gonorrhea, herpes, syphilis, pubic lice, HIV, trichomonas, and HPV. Some symptoms of an STI include: sores or bumps on the genitals or in the oral or rectal area, painful or burning urination, discharge from the penis, unusual or odd-smelling vaginal discharge and/or vaginal bleeding, and pain during sex. It is important to note that many STIs have no symptoms at all, which is why it is essential to get tested regularly.

was my job to organize literature and videos about sexuality and disease. Single fathers came in to check out materials on sex education and would ask me how to talk to their teenage daughters about sex. At high school parties and during recess, other kids sought me out with questions about urinary tract infections, blow jobs, and birth control. My advice of drinking cranberry juice to clear up UTIs had the additional effect of clearing the urine of marijuana traces. This made me popular with peers who wanted to beat drug tests. There were many times when the topics at hand were beyond my skill set. It was the early 1990s, so we didn't have Google to look up "how to give the best blow job" or "can you get an STI from anal sex?" Even the staff on-site at Planned Parenthood weren't prepared to answer the more personal and emotional questions my friends and I had about sex.

I knew that one day there just HAD to be a centralized place to find all the latest and greatest information on sex and deliver it in an approachable, mindful way. And, taking a cue from my recess days, I knew I needed to create it.

Hence, The Sex Ed was born.

I founded TheSexEd.com platform and *The Sex Ed* podcast in 2018, with a core philosophy: *pleasure and sexual health are essential not only to surviving but to thriving.* I believe we need to consider our sexuality holistically and apply now commonly accepted mindfulness techniques to the way we think about, talk about, educate about, and have sex.

We might believe we have invented the wheel when it comes to sex, but almost everything you can think of has been around in one form or another since the dawn of humanity. The act of sex wasn't all that different centuries ago.

The oldest known stone phallus—which looks a lot like a dildo, although it may in fact be an object of ritual worship—is about twenty-seven to twenty-eight thousand years old. Now Bluetooth technology has given us remote-controlled sex toys and pleasure robots. (Human desires don't change much; technology does.) What has remained mostly consistent in all these thousands of years is a spiritual estrangement between our consciousness and the way we approach sexuality. My life mission is to change that. We tend to disassociate our body, and particularly our genitals, from our mind and soul—siloing sex into a narrow box that doesn't allow us to fully express ourselves or tap into the awesome power of sexuality as a source of energy and creativity.

We absorb shame around our bodies and our primal feelings from the time we are little kids, instead of receiving the message that desire is okay and that there are healthy ways to set boundaries around it. Instead of learning to be comfortable first and foremost with our own sexuality, bodies, and desires, we are taught to measure our worth, validity, and desirability through the eyes of others.

How are we meant to align and integrate our understanding of sex, health, and consciousness in a culture where "sex ed" is now mostly gleaned via streaming porn, without our being given the tools to decipher what we are taking in?

Consider this book a radical imagining of Sex Ed 101. Together, we are going to dismantle everything we *thought* we knew about sex in order to build a new foundation. One that is based on the awareness that sex, health, and consciousness intersect to form our understanding of ourselves and sexuality. I'm here to teach you that sexuality and spirituality *do* intersect—and, in turn, that the connection between the two will lead you to a healthier, more sexually empowered life. Through this process of reprogramming and reclaiming what this word *sex* means, we will discover how to be more authentic, experience greater pleasure, and have more enlightened relationships with ourselves and our lovers!

Ever since I was a teenager, I imagined a time in the future when I would have it all figured out. I would know who I was and be completely at ease in my skin. I wouldn't question myself or encounter anxiety, depression, or insecurity. Life would be smooth.

I spent years watching friends, family, mentors, and people I admired from afar, wishing I was as self-assured, secure, successful, happy in relationships, or "together" as they were. I wanted to know their secrets. How could I become the healthy, confident, sexually empowered woman that I wanted to be? How should I navigate my relationships in a new frontier of sexual/gender roles and rules? How best should I care for my health, body, and mind?

A researcher by nature, I turned to experts.

Research has always been a refuge for me—a place where I could tune out uncertainty and fears, getting lost in piles of paper, stacks of books, and my wild imagination.

As a young married woman, I was an anomaly among my friends and peers, due to being in a monogamous relationship throughout my twenties and also as someone who investigated sexuality professionally. At eighteen, while studying photography at the School of Visual Arts in New York City, I had started collecting burlesque costumes at flea markets. As part of a thesis project for school, I photographed myself in the costumes, attempting to emulate the glamour poses of the great burlesque queens of the 1930s and '40s. I wanted to look like they did: strong women who appeared empowered by their sexuality. I was still bewildered by my own.

I tracked down the last surviving twentieth-century American burlesque queens and recorded their first-person stories, spending time with them at their homes, businesses, and hospital rooms at the end of their lives. I learned firsthand the lost art of burlesque as they dressed me in their old costumes and taught me trademark moves. Some of the queens had wanted to be in showbiz; some had been abused; some had exchanged sexual favors offstage for extra cash. All had a lot to tell me about sex, heterosexual men, and how stripping affected their psyche. In a sense, I had my first sexual awakening as a married woman via eighty-year-old strippers passing their hard-earned wisdom down to me.

I directed a documentary about my experiences, *Pretty Things* (HBO, 2005) and wrote a book, *Pretty Things: The Last Generation of American Burlesque Queens* (HarperCollins, 2006). As I was finishing up a book tour, my marriage slowly began to unravel, a process that took a couple of years. I realized that I still had a lot to learn about who I was and what I wanted out of life, let alone a relationship.

While exploring my sexuality and new relationships postdivorce, I was also delving into academic archives and libraries in search of information on late nineteenth-century prostitutes, pimps, and madams for a second book, *Sporting Guide: Los Angeles, 1897* (Regan Arts, 2015), set in the world of vice and sex work.

As I analyzed 1840–1910 census records, making notes for my book, I was also conducting first-person research—falling in and out of love and trying experiences on for size. I questioned my personal network of "sexperts" and friends about how best to navigate sex and dating in my thirties. I was often struck by the parallels between the nineteenth century and the present day; the human experience of love, grief, and sex remains unchanged by time.

In 2012, a friend, the adult film star and author Nina Hartley, invited me to sit in on her guest lecture for a sex education, therapy, and behavior seminar at the University of California, Los Angeles. When I arrived, the previous lecturers, an adult film actress and producer, were finishing their presentation and handing out research materials—their pornographic DVDs—to the students, an eager crowd of licensed and practicing sex therapists and medical residents.

The professor of the class, the late Walter Brackelmanns, was director of the couples and sex training program. He had been teaching at UCLA for fifty years and was president and cofounder of the American Association of Couples and Sex Therapists. Meeting Walter and his codirector, Wendy Cherry, felt like landing in sex-ed heaven. Dr. Brackelmanns and Dr. Cherry welcomed me into the seminar, which I audited (and eventually guest lectured in myself) for many years to follow. They became mentors, colleagues, and friends.

I've now spent close to three decades exploring sexuality, both professionally and personally. Every experience in my private life, as well as all my academic and anecdotal research, has cemented my belief that integrating mind, body, and spirit is essential for sexual wellness.

I've interviewed doctors, professors, scientists, and practitioners in the fields of mental and physical health, sexuality, bondage, yoga, meditation, and space exploration. I've recorded conversations with a wide range of friends, including surfers, high school students, botanists, historians, cultural practitioners, and sex workers. In the process I have received loads of helpful, practical advice on sexuality, health, and consciousness. Everyone had something useful to share.

I found that happiness and pleasure are not out of reach. We all have the ability to accept and love ourselves exactly as we are, in the moment we are in, flaws and all.

So why do we have so much trouble doing so?

Is it because our culture doesn't teach us at an early age to celebrate and cherish our bodies, our sexuality, and our mental wellness? Is it because there are so many easy opportunities to tear ourselves and others down instead of being kind and loving?

Why is it that when we feel our lowest, we look outside for assurance? We seek validation or escape in someone or something else—sex, food, drugs, alcohol, electronic devices. Not that there's anything wrong with healthy escapism or a vice or two, but it's easy to fall down the rabbit hole of self-destructive behavior and then feel shame over whatever it is we "shouldn't" be doing. Why can't we be gentler on ourselves?

I longed for a guidebook on how to handle my challenging times—divorce at thirty-one to a man I had met at eighteen; PTSD from multiple traumas; the illness and death of my father. I remember during a particularly low point asking one of my best friends how long it would take to feel better and being frustrated by her answer: "It will just take as long as it takes." I wanted a magic pill to cure my loneliness, insecurity, heartbreak, and grief.

I decided to approach each difficult moment as an opportunity to change myself, my attitude, my life. After my divorce, I moved into the first apartment I'd ever had on my own and drank my morning tea with our wedding china. I fell in and out of love again. I started meditating. I took risks in my career. I redefined my relationship to my sexuality. I learned patience, trust, and forgiveness. I spent as much time with my dying father as I could, to hold on to every bit of him.

I realized that people come into our lives to love, hurt, teach, leave, and heal us. That situations occur to offer us lessons. That nobody has it any more figured out than anybody else. Most importantly, that being truly *conscious* of my desires, boundaries, relationships, and sexuality comes with the reward of a more fulfilling sex life.

The amazing thing is that we hold all the mysteries of the universe within us. But somewhere along the way, we stopped listening to our instinct and intuition. We forgot how to have self-love, self-esteem, and self-acceptance.

I don't claim to be an ultimate guru on sex, health, and consciousness. You are ultimately your own best guide! But real life and professional research have given me tools and experienced authorities to call upon when I am struggling. I wrote this book to share the practical advice I have gathered along the way. And to remind myself—and all of you—that we don't need to have it all together all of the time in order to awaken the guru inherent inside all of us.

So how does this relate back to sex, you ask?

Let's start with a simple exercise.

Close your eyes and take a deep breath in. Hold your breath in for three counts and then slowly exhale, allowing your belly to fully release. Great. Now do it again twice more. Feeling settled? Now let's do it again, but as you exhale, bring your focus to your genitals. Notice how they feel—itchy? Wet? Dry? Sticky? Tingly? Numb? Whatever adjective you choose to describe the current state of affairs down below is okay! Just noticing and naming it is the first step on the road to a marvelous new relationship with your sexual health.

With your eyes still closed, breathe again deeply, exhaling all the way down your throat, chest, and belly and into your genitals. Do this slowly with me now, three times in a row. Do you feel any change in sensation? Are there any new adjectives you'd like to add to your list? Does it make you uncomfortable or feel awkward, weird, stupid, shameful, scary, silly, exciting, or titillating to check in with your penis or vagina?

Still with me?

The first step is becoming *aware*. Applying our *consciousness*, remember?

So much of what drives us has to do with sex and relationships. We also tend to define ourselves and others by sexual standards that equate sex with self-worth. Add social media and the ready availability of porn to the mix and it is easy to see why our current culture tends to view sex as transactional, detached from spirituality and a higher state of consciousness.

Let's get a few basic truths straight.

Sex is not an act for which you need another person to participate in.

Sex doesn't need to culminate in orgasm to be a powerful experience or "good."

Sex affects every single area of your life, including your decision-making process, whether or not you compartmentalize it.

Your sexual energy is one and the same as your creative energy. (Yogis and Eastern cultures often refer to this as "prana," "qi," etc.) Athletes and artists (among them supposedly William Shakespeare and Mae West) often abstained from partnered sex when training for a big game or completing a creative work.

If we can expand our ideas of what sex and our sexuality are and have the potential to be, we can begin to tap into them as sources of power and personal growth.

I would much rather be having consciousness-altering, transcendent sex and exist in a society that values and honors a full spectrum of sexuality and gender identity. I want to live in a culture that is actively removing shame, fear, trauma, and taboos around sex and normalizing an integrative, expansive approach to human sexuality.

So how do we achieve this? By creating a new archetype for sex education, one that is based on the alignment of *sex, health, and consciousness*. In order for you to have the best relationship with your sexuality—and, therefore, the best sex possible—we need to make sure your mind, body, and consciousness are calibrated and operating in equilibrium.

Getting clear on how we approach each of these areas personally *and* how to integrate them are the foundations needed to reach truly transcendent sex— and what you'll learn in this book. A simple analogy to explain my philosophy is to the chakra system. In lay terms, chakras are energy centers located throughout your body, from the base of your spine all the way up to the top of your head. Think of them as your energetic nervous system. From bottom to top, these chakras are:

Root: located at the base of your spine around the perineum
Sacral: located just below the navel
Solar: located around your abdomen below the uppermost rib
Heart: located at your heart
Throat: located at your throat
Third eye: located in between your eyebrows
Crown: located at the top of your head

We'll be examining sexual wellness from the ground, or root, up. First, we'll be exploring our sense of safety (our root chakra) and sex (our sacral chakra) as a foundation. What is our current understanding of sex, intimacy, and pleasure? What societal "norms" have been ingrained in us that prevent us from being comfortable with ourselves? What traumas must we confront, communicate about, and honor in order to have a better relationship with ourselves and our partners? Starting at the root and sacral chakras will challenge us to throw out everything we've been taught and to redefine our version of normal.

Without having a real understanding of these fundamental parts of our being, we can't move on to the second aspect we look at in this book: health. This segment of the book explores our center, or the solar plexus and heart chakras, which shape how we view ourselves, our self-esteem, our level of confidence, and our relationships with others. Working with our center makes us examine everything: how we use sex in our lives, what our deepest desires are, even how we experience and express love.

Finally, we get to consciousness, located in our upper chakras—the throat, third eye, and crown. After we have reflected on our sexuality and wellness, becoming more aware and secure in ourselves and our needs, we can move on to look at how we communicate, trust, and use our intuition to tune in to our higher selves. Consciousness is our invitation to play!

Consciousness cannot exist without a total understanding of sex and health. Imagine all seven of these chakras as a set of well-lubed golden wheels, each ideally spinning in the same direction at the same speed. Our experiences, relationships, family histories, and cultural and religious backgrounds all play a part in how these wheels function individually and as a whole. If there is trauma, shame, excess, fear, or lack of education around one area (for example, a culturally learned idea that menstruation is gross, dirty, and unsexy), it can throw off our whole system, impacting our sense of self-worth (we feel gross, dirty, and unsexy) and how we experience sex (we avoid period sex and miss out on the benefits of orgasming to relieve cramps!).

We are so culturally wired toward instant gratification that we want to skip the steps and get to the end result, like, NOW! I get asked all the time for quick tantra tips, and my answer tends to frustrate those who would rather take a pill or watch a short YouTube tutorial—you gotta do the work from the ground up in order to achieve the most transformative results.

The exciting (and sometimes challenging) thing about our sexuality is that no two of us are alike. Each of us has a sexual identity that is like a thumbprint—completely unique. None of us will experience sexuality or identify exactly the same way. We are also constantly evolving from the time we come onto the planet until we leave it, including in the ways we relate to ourselves and others sexually. This book and The Sex Ed platform are here to help you (and me!) figure out how to be comfortable with our bodies, how to love, and how we like to fuck at each stage of our lives.

One of the biggest challenges we face on our sexual journey is to let go of what we *think* we know, like, or believe about sex. This includes our snap judgments, inherent biases, and cultural conditioning around shame and taboo. I am not promising you that it will be easy—this book doesn't wrap up sex in a neat millennial-pink package and remove the awkwardness and gray areas that come with the topic. You may find sexual fetishes or lifestyles discussed within these pages that make you truly uncomfortable. But if you are committed to learning (and to continuing after you finish reading), I promise to help open you up to possibilities of pleasure you may have never thought to explore before.

I want to provide you with power: the power to make informed decisions, to enlarge your sexual repertoire, to say no or yes, to have better orgasms—even to expand your spiritual consciousness through integrative awareness of your body and sexuality.

When it comes to sexuality, there's always more to learn. More education and communication around intimacy and sex lead to a healthier culture and healthier self. I believe we stand at the threshold of entering into a new sexual paradigm that will greatly expand our ability to align more truthfully with our deepest desires—all of which will allow us to better embody *pleasure.*

So let's throw out everything you've learned about sex and lay the groundwork for a *more orgasmic, more mind-blowing, more fulfilling, more authentic experience of your own sexual health and consciousness.* None of this is going to be easy. I don't care what celebs, tech gurus, or spiritual healers promise, there is no such thing as a quick-fix workshop, plant medicine journey, or deep prayer that then results in us being all "healed." It is a lifelong process to align our sex, health, and consciousness. There will be times when our old programming and stories rear their heads. These moments will require being gentle with yourself. It is okay to hold grief for our old ways and simultaneously keep faith in the new.

A few key things to remember as we embark on this journey:

YOU are the master of your pleasure.
YOU are the master of your healing.
YOU are the master of experiencing divine love, sex, and intimacy.

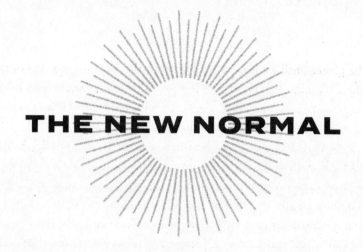

THE NEW NORMAL

Do you remember how old you were when you first heard the word *normal* spoken in conjunction with sex, body type, genitalia, desire, relationships, love, or behavior? Did you hear it from your parents, through media, or from friends? Can you go way back in your memories to locate where your definition of normal was established?

We all have a different version of what we consider normal, depending on where and how we grew up, the standards for beauty and behavior that were modeled to us from an early age, and how we consumed this information. It is highly doubtful that any of us used critical thinking to examine whether these messages around "normalcy" were accurate. Instead, we accepted that there was an "expected" or "typical" body size, sexual desire, physical and emotional development process, and so forth to conform to.

It's strange that regardless of who we are and where we come from, we all have been trained to measure up to a standardized "norm." If we each see colors a different way (what I call blue you might label turquoise, teal, or violet) and we all have unique fingerprints (and sexual identities), then why are we using the same reference point for what is normal?

Instead of building our own references for what normal means to each of us, we unconsciously learn to measure ourselves against others and against cultural expectations when it comes to sexuality, love, and our own bodies. And we do it *constantly.*

What if we decided to throw out this invisible barometer of "normal" and learned how to be truly comfortable with our sexuality, bodies, feelings, and desires? Our bodies and brains are all wired individually, and each of us has novel benchmarks for growth, body shape, and stimulation. Outside influences are what make us place value, judgment, and shame on ourselves and how "normal" we are.

Sadly, shame has been an essential part of how we learn about sexuality and what we determine to be "normal." From the time we are little, sex and our bodies cause us so many feelings of humiliation, distress, and foolishness. We become stuck in an endless loop of judging ourselves and others based on what we think is "correct"—that is, won't cause us embarrassment or make us stand out from the "norm."

It is extremely confusing to figure out our true normal baseline, or what is correct for us as individuals, in a culture that doesn't provide access to real information about sex, relationship negotiations, communication, or desire. Mostly we are given explicit images via porn without the emotional tools to decipher them; taught body shame from an early age, often unintentionally, by our family and peers; and force-fed images by mass media and literature that reinforce uniform ideals to aspire to.

When was the first time you had a conscious ideal of what was "normal" for dick size or for when to have sex? Many boys grow up learning through pop-culture mythology and porn that their penis length should be around seven to eight inches. Statistically, a more accurate average would be around five to five and a half inches. Is anyone pointing that out to them? Or to sexual partners who are judging them by these guidelines? If we consider that most, if not all, of early sexual activity—and this includes masturbation and experimenting sexually with friends—occurs with zero communication (and often in secret), how are we meant to untangle the myriad lies around "normal" that we've been conditioned to accept?

All of this comparing and despairing[3] as we measure ourselves against "normal" creates massive internalized shame that suffocates us. This shame holds us back from being the most fully realized, joyful, and orgasmic versions of ourselves.

Let's unpack the normal we have been using as our standard.

When you decided what was normal, did you compare yourself to your friends' bodies? To movie stars or athletes? To porn stars? To the Kardashians? Did you feel ashamed because you thought your pussy/dick/tits/ass was too small/big/hairy/not hairy? Did you worry that your body or sexuality didn't measure up to the norm? Whom did you talk to about all these insecurities?

---

3   If you were born after 1994, the internet and social media have likely made your sense of compare and despair about ten billion times higher than it was for previous generations.

I certainly didn't ask my parents if I was normal or if it was okay to masturbate or whether my body was desirable. As a kid, I was never told that it was normal and healthy to masturbate, that my body was beautiful, or that I'd be better off not comparing myself to other people's physiologies and sexual development.

When did you first learn about puberty, menstruation, pubic hair, ejaculation, blow jobs, and genital hygiene? Did someone sit you down and have a "talk" with you? Maybe you were handed a couple of graphic novels by Peter Mayle, like I was—*Where Did I Come From?*, which covered how babies are born, and *What's Happening to Me?*, about adolescence. I remember looking at the comic illustrations by Arthur Robins in those books, comparing myself to the images of developing body parts, wondering when my breasts would warrant a training bra and if my vagina was growing at the right speed.

Nick Kroll, cocreator and writer of the Emmy-nominated animated Netflix series *Big Mouth*, about the awkward stages of puberty, told me these books also made a big impact on his childhood—enough so to influence his writing of the characters on his show. Nick said, **"We have What's Happening to Me? in our office, and I just looked at it like, 'Oh, wow.' These books were formative for me of like, okay, that's where his penis is at that age, in that sort of progression from child to adolescent to young man to man to old man, and I remember clocking all of that on men and women and being like, 'Where do I fall on all this?'"**

We aren't taught as kids that our desires are okay or how to set boundaries around our bodies and desires. So is it any wonder we have a world full of screwed-up adults struggling to connect and make sense of their own sexuality, let alone find love, healthy relationships, and great sex with others?

Most general-use sex books available prior to 2016, sex-ed curricula (if available), and medical textbooks—in fact, the entire medical system—are based on a patriarchal,[4] white supremacist,[5] heteronormative, binary model of gender and sex. Intercourse has been depicted and referred to as occurring only between a man and a woman for the purpose of procreation; in this paradigm, there exist only two genders and ways of identifying.

---

4   This term refers to the societal prevalence of cis-male-dominant social norms. These manifest in cis men occupying leadership roles in political, religious, professional, academic, and familial contexts (among others) and have historically led to the second-class citizenship of anyone perceived to be non–cis male within many facets of culture and experience.

5   The belief and ideology that upholds Eurocentric whiteness as being above, or superior to, all other racial and ethnic groups. Much of Western culture has been built upon this principle.

The (old) "normal" sexual framework most of us grew up under and are still operating within doesn't account for, let alone understand, how to support anyone who doesn't fit in a narrow metric: Man. Woman. Fuck. Missionary.

Truth is, gender and sexual identification exist along a massive spectrum. Viewing our gender and sexual identities through a restrictive lens prevents us from allowing these identities to be fluid and evolving. They're not like filling out a medical intake or census form with limited boxes to check. I may currently identify as a heterosexual woman, but how does that allow for my being attracted to women? Do I consider myself 100 percent straight? No, and often people (usually hetero) who are forceful in asserting that they are 100 percent on one end of the spectrum are fighting against internalized repression and fear that their identity may be more gray than they would like to acknowledge. If we try to fit our uniqueness into a neat little box that makes it easier for other people or the wider culture to label and therefore "understand" us, we are confining ourselves within an ideology that doesn't work in the first place.

I say, *fuck the old normal*. If it had been working for any of us, there would be no market for self-help, spirituality, or improve-your-sexual-and-emotional-health books like this one.

The (old) "normal" was built upon patriarchal, white supremacist ideals that allowed reproductive health advances to be linked to nonconsensual use of enslaved people and free black women as "research subjects." Scratch the surface of the "father of modern gynecology" and inventor of the speculum, the white American physician James Marion Sims, and you will uncover a man who performed genital surgeries on black women without anesthesia in the name of "medicine." One of his "patients" was purported to have been operated on three hundred times before she died. Infant mortality, high-risk pregnancy, and reproductive health issues for black mothers continue to be a massive problem (particularly in the United States) to this day.

The (old) "normal" for what Western culture held as an "ideal" body type was also dictated according to white supremacy—whether we consider the voluptuous nudes of the Italian Renaissance (painted by white Europeans) or Barbie's "perfect" bust-waist-hip measurements (thirty-six, twenty-four, thirty-six inches). When it comes to the ways in which nonwhite female bodies have been eroticized, exploited, and often rejected by Western culture, one must familiarize oneself with the dark story of the "Hottentot

Venus." In the early nineteenth century, Alexander Dunlop, a military surgeon in a Cape Town slave lodge, had a side hustle of supplying showbiz exhibitors in the United Kingdom with animal specimens. He coerced and captured a South African Khoikhoi woman (alternately known as Sarah or Saartjie Baartman) to put her on display. She was exhibited to the public, wearing very little clothing, for the perverse thrill of European onlookers and scientists intent on "studying" her body curves and labia folds. She died after five years of being subjected to these horrific "studies" at the hands of men. Upon her death in France, Baartman's remains (and specifically her sexual organs) were subjected to a lurid postmortem, as further examples of "scientific interest." It was only in 2002, more than two hundred years after Sarah's birth, that France finally returned her remains so her bones could be laid to rest in her homeland. So no, we haven't come a long way, baby. In fact, we are only at the beginning of reexamining most of the history, scientific, and medical textbooks that we take as "fact."

It is demanding to establish a good relationship with our sexuality when our basic self-esteem has been linked to comparing ourselves with the products of a broken system and other people's experiences of puberty and sex. When we examine what have been considered "normal" sex, love, genitalia, and human physiques for thousands of years, we also have to ask who defined these ideas of "normal" and whom these ideas serve.

Before we blame our parents, grandparents, religion, or cultural background for what we perceive to be a lack of or detrimental education around sex, we should remember that it's highly unlikely any of them had the tools themselves to communicate in a healthy way around these subjects.

Let's take the premise that everything we have learned about sex so far comes from people and organizations that either shroud self-pleasure and sex outside of marriage in shame, fear, and taboo or aren't licensed sexologists, therapists, or sex educators. If we start from that assumption, then we have to *question everything* we take as gospel.

The collective baggage we have around sexuality goes back so far—literally, centuries—that we need to throw out all our preconceived notions and biases about what we think is "normal" when it comes to our desires or inhibitions, and we must begin anew.

I spend 80 percent of my time on The Sex Ed responding to people around the world wanting to know some version of whether their body, desires, fluids (or lack thereof), or sexual experiences are "normal." These questions can include anything from concerns whether there is a "right" size for vulvas or penises (There is no such thing. Yours is perfect, and as long as you love it, someone else in the world will, too) to if it is "normal" to lose desire in a long-term relationship. (Yes, absolutely, you need to put effort into your sex life if you want it to improve, kind of like you have to train for a marathon. I like to tell people to schedule sex or even makeout sessions as a regular discipline. It's hot to send your partner an iCal reminder to fuck. Get creative.) And on the kinkier side, there are just as many "Will others think I am normal?" questions.

Here are my takeaways from being on the receiving end of these kinds of questions every day:

1. We all seem to be subliminally measuring ourselves against a standard for "normal" or sexual gold medal winners.

2. We equate "normal" with "good." How and when did we set this standard for "normal"? Who is this imaginary person who always has mind-blowing, perfect sex and whose body always performs perfectly? Are we comparing ourselves to what we see in the media (fantasy) or in porn (more fantasy)? Maybe we think our friends' experiences are the "normal" we should be trying to achieve?

3. We are so worried about what other people think and our own internalized shame that we stop ourselves from being the real freak in the sheets that we want to be.

We need to go back to the beginning to figure out whether our patterns and belief systems are *actually* working for us. Then we need to reprogram, reparent, and reclaim ourselves in order to experience real sexual freedom. Put yourself in the mindset of a kid just beginning to read. It's a little challenging, sometimes frustrating, but also exciting, because you can't wait to get to the juicy big-kid books. But first you gotta master the ABCs.

Each of us has a endless erotic library to explore (one of my personal fantasies), and we are going to start together at the first stack by redefining what is "normal" when it comes to sexuality. There are a few ABSOLUTE HARD NO's when it comes to "normal":

1. You do not have sex with anyone without their consent.

2. You do not have sex with minors, dead people, or animals—none of whom can grant consent.

3. You do not engage in abusive sexual or violent behavior.

Outside of the aforementioned hard no's, 99 percent of humans on this planet (myself included) want to be reassured that they are not alone in their experience or insecurities. You would be surprised how common (indeed, normal) your neuroses are once you start receiving the volume of messages I do. Many other people on the planet are asking the *exact same* question that you are right at this very moment! If you think you are the only person with a pie, foot, diaper, prosthetic leg, or [insert yours here] fetish, spend some time on FetLife, a.k.a. Tinder/Grindr, for the fetish and kink community.

Human sexuality is ever evolving. What fascinates us about bodies and sex as teenagers is different from what draws us when we are in our twenties, thirties, forties, and eighties. And remember, we each have a unique sexual identity. No two people are alike. So we have to throw out the idea of "normal" and give up judging how much or what kind of sex we are having in comparison to another. (PS Everyone lies.)

Even someone like me who spends most of their day talking, reading, and writing about sex has to face up to what I think "normal" is. Most people expect me, as a sex-positive sex researcher and historian, to have a superwild personal life. One close friend told me that the first time she came to my house, she expected me to answer the door wearing animal print while swinging from the ceiling. While I believe animal print is a neutral and I do have a penchant for swings, I am much more the 1950s monogamous housewife archetype, happiest in a committed partnership, cooking dinner and cutting roses at home in lingerie, rather than wilding out with casual sex and multiple lovers.

The first person I ever slept with on the first night we met, I ended up marrying. Granted, I was eighteen and had had less than a handful of sexual partners at the time, but I never got better at separating sex from love.

When my marriage was nearing an end after thirteen years (spanning my twenties, when everyone I knew was out screwing everyone else I knew), I was so deeply unhappy and lonely that I thought the answer was to open up the marriage sexually. I was committed to my wedding vows and to our promise of sexual monogamy, but at the same time I was searching for a way to ask my husband for permission to sleep with other people. I even had someone in mind, someone who had made it clear he had romantic feelings for me. Although I hadn't crossed a physical line, I was getting close.

My husband and I were coming home from seeing a band play at the Troubadour in West Hollywood one night, talking about what a good show it was. And in particular, how the lead singers were husband and wife. He mentioned that they were swingers. I perked up, asking lots of questions, eventually getting the courage to blurt out, "So what do you think of that?" He stopped at a red light, turned to me in the car, looked me straight in the eye, and said, "I would be okay with you sleeping with other men if it would save our marriage."

It shut me up. I realized I wanted intimacy, partnership, and love, too. I wasn't going to be fulfilled by the quick fix of having someone else inside of me. It was a much deeper problem I had to solve.

When we divorced, everyone was shocked that he and I had been monogamous for all that time. I can't count how many times I heard, "You gotta get under someone to get over someone." Oh, how I would try!

Why couldn't I be the kind of woman who was joyfully polyamorous or had a domestic submissive to pick up my laundry and clean my dishes? Why did I hold back from every one of the supersexy top female porn stars who wanted to get to know me better? I was jealous of friends who regaled me with stories of abandon and lust with a stranger. I love a good porn story line, but every time I would see someone and think, "I want to fuck them," I'd end up in a relationship within weeks.

A few months into a committed relationship, after I was hooked on the sex high, I would willfully ignore the signals from my heart and head—*this is not aligned with what you want in a partner, Liz*—and instead try to mold the sexual relationship to meet my committed-partnership expectations. My inability to compartmentalize my sexuality and my heart allowed my libido to get the best of me again and again, always with the same disappointing results.

A fast fuck with a stranger sounds hot when I fantasize about it—but I'm someone who doesn't even let people wear shoes in my house. I am so sensitive to other people's energy that I just can't help but confuse sex with emotional and romantic attachment, even when I know better. It took me a long time (truthfully, within relationships during my thirties and early forties) to understand my boundaries and deepest wishes around sex and love.

In order to get to this place, I had to stop comparing myself to the "norm," which is the opposite of what I truly desire for myself. I used to be insecure about having such old-fashioned personal ideals of monogamy. Given what I do for a living and the high percentage of sexual and gender fluidity within my peer group, I often felt like a prude. That is, until I gave up comparing my sex life with anyone other than myself.

Nina Hartley has perhaps the longest-running career of any woman in the adult industry. As a longtime performer of sex acts on and off camera, Nina has already had more sex with more people than most of us will in our lifetime. She identifies as "quite kinky" and has been in dominant/submissive, poly, and queer partnerships . . . yet she told me that she was envious of my ability to have multiple orgasms! So there you go. Even the people you think have the sexual gold medals fall into the trap of comparing and despairing.

A new normal widens the current definition of sex beyond the narrow requirement of penetration and an orgasmic outcome. Sex can be making out, licking, stroking, spanking, fingering—so many flavors—and intimacy and pleasure can be cultivated in all these acts as well.

A new normal allows you to define the perimeter of your sandbox and the toys you'd like to play with, understanding that at any point you can toss out a toy that no longer suits you and try something new. And no, I don't mean toys as in other people—playing with people sexually and discarding them is bad sexual etiquette, not to mention unkind.

If you open up beyond the current constrictions that you, family, society, and/or religion place on your erotic dreams, you may discover you have a penchant for shrimping (sucking on toes) or love getting a cream pie in the face or feel a thrill being spanked with a flogger or having your corset tightly laced. There is a high probability that you haven't scratched the surface of what your kinks may be. Isn't it exciting that you have the rest of your life to discover and rediscover and discover again what turns you on? It's like going into an ice cream shop with ten million choices and toppings—think of all the sweet, creamy treats to taste!

Sexuality is a personal journey. What works for me, Nina, him, or them may not float your boat. It is vital to be comfortable with your own desires, first and foremost. It is also important to make sure that when you decide to try something new sexually, you are deciding for yourself and not being coaxed into it. Discuss it with someone you trust, apart from your partner, if you are not sure. Negotiate consent before, during, and after a new experience. These are all intricate parts of having a sexual encounter. *Sex doesn't happen perfectly and mysteriously, like in the movies, and talking about it beforehand doesn't make it less sexy.*

A new normal includes self-esteem, boundaries, and clear communication around sex. A new normal discourages our current standard of having mostly disassociative sex, with our body disengaged from our mind and heart. A new normal integrates our spirituality and consciousness with our sexuality. A new normal encourages play!

I like to live my life with the attitude that I may join the circus one day in my seventies. So while I have certain hard no's, I'm open to talking about my own and my partner's fantasies before I decide whether I want to try something new sexually. As we evolve, our desires do as well.

Asa Akira is a legendary porn star, director, author, and podcaster. She has performed in more than five hundred films, is known as the "Anal Queen," and in 2013 became the third Asian person ever to win the AVN Female Performer of the Year award given by *Adult Video News*. She told me, that **"on a personal level, my sexual tastes are ever evolving. I used to think that sexual preference or sexual taste was a thing you're born with, and that's it. Since being in porn, I've found that it's not the case. Sometimes it evolves in one direction, and then it reverts back. It's okay to change your mind about things or have a flavor of the week. I'm learning that's okay and normal, rather than pigeonholing myself into one thing as if it's what I have to like forever."**

Another thing to consider in our new normal is this: *monogamy is not a natural state for humans but a matter of choice.* Much like virginity, it is a societal construct we have developed over thousands of years of evolution and a convenience for the benefit of people and systems in places of power. It may be what works for me or you, or it may not—but if it is the accepted cultural standard for committed relationships, we need to be aware that we are constantly fighting against our basic primal instinct. There are so many options and conversations to have with yourself and your partners to decide what works best for you.

The cool part of where we are right *now* in terms of culture, technology, history, and advances in health is that so many of us are questioning the relationship structures we have been told are normal and figuring out new language and parameters for building new kinds of intimate partnerships.

For example, let's take polyamory, which is the practice of engaging in multiple *consensual* romantic, sexual, or intimate relationships. This can also be called consensual nonmonogamy or an open relationship—the terminology is constantly changing as the old systems get torn down and recreated. Couples in such relationships often establish explicit boundaries (regarding frequency, specific acts, disclosure, etc.) in order to preserve the comfort of the primary partner within the agreement. I know many polyamorous couples in kink- or fetish-based relationships who are successful in managing expectations and evolving desires because they have the basis for a more open dialogue around sex and intimacy.

Outside of sex-positive and kink communities, though, this word often gets bandied about without all of its parameters and boundaries being acknowledged. I regularly have women in their twenties ask me about polyamory after being introduced to the concept by a hipster partner who views it as an opportunity to get more pussy "ethically." Winston Wilde, a kink-aware therapist, asks young patients who come into his office wanting to try polyamory, "Have you ever had a relationship with one person? Master that first—it's hard enough."

I am not making the case that polyamory is a more evolved lifestyle than monogamy, only that all of these options are choices and are, indeed, normal. We need to understand what relationship dynamics work for us, talk about it with our partners, and check in repeatedly—our criteria for what we need is going to change as we do, and so will theirs.

Kenneth Play is a sex educator and sex coach who has been called "the world's greatest sex hacker" by *GQ* magazine. He also identifies as polyamorous. Kenneth says, **"I think the misconception is that if you are poly you are never jealous, you never need alone time, you never need one on one, you never need devotion. I think all those desires still exist in people. I think nonmonogamy just offers some more flexibility and possibility on how to engineer it. It's more like designing and learning and seeing what fits all the individuals in the relationship."**

You have the freedom to choose different relationship paradigms for the different people who come into your life and at different stages of *your* evolution.

A new normal includes embracing and celebrating the awkward, messy *humanness* of our own bodies—our genitals, reproductive systems, noises, fluids, and smells. Contrary to what so many companies push, vaginas are self-cleaning and do not need to be douched with harsh irritants; ultimately what is being sold is a historical myth that they are "unclean." Many of our longstanding cultural beliefs about menstruation have caused us to have deep shame, whether we are the ones menstruating or not! Our new normal also doesn't send us into a spiral of, yep, you guessed it, shame when we have trouble getting an erection or ejaculating or getting wet—because there are about a thousand different factors that could be playing into each of these scenarios. They are all normal, and we don't need to blame our inner selves for our physiology not functioning according to some ideal of perfection all the time.

Now that we understand that our foundational ideas about sexuality have some shortcomings, the next step is to rebuild one that works for you, dear reader. Each of our rebuilt foundations will be different while also respectful of each other's.

We are going to replace our old answers and thoughts with new ones that will serve us better. At the end of this chapter, I will offer an exercise to help you to create *your new normal.* In order to do this, first we need to take an *objective, detached, honest* look at ourselves and throw out a couple of things that are holding us back:

1. The old normal: See it in the rearview mirror. Acknowledge it is not working, or you wouldn't be reading this book. The old normal will still trip us up sometimes, but that is okay—your sexual evolution has a learning curve, and no one expects you to be perfect, know all the latest nomenclature for gender and sexual identities, or be up to date on current research, news, and sexual trends. I encourage you to lean into education if you don't know something or want to understand yourself better. People all around the world are using The Sex Ed as a resource for the same purposes. And no, I don't think you (or I for that matter) should have it all figured out by now.

2. Shame: We learn to carry shame early. It defines the way we feel about ourselves and how we relate to our body, our sexuality, our love patterns, and our relationships. We have to go way back and figure out what experiences made us feel mortified, degraded, cut down to size, humiliated, debased, unloved, unwanted, abandoned, or left lacking. Our shame is a big part of what is holding us back from creating amazing intimate and sexual relationships with ourselves and others.

Does any of this sound easy? NO! It's work! Where did we get this idea that we are just supposed to be "good" at sex without any effort? Do you make time to exercise, meditate, eat well, sleep enough, hydrate? Why not be as disciplined about discovering what gives you pleasure? Sex is a lifetime adventure, and part of our new normal is a recognition that we don't know what we don't know—plus a commitment to be willing to learn, right?

As the seminal Parliament-Funkadelic sophomore album title suggests: *Free Your Mind . . . and Your Ass Will Follow.* Let's stay in that mindset as we each develop our new normal, starting with digging through the old programming that is holding us back from our potential as authentic, fulfilled sexual beings. Here is an exercise that will help you do just that.

1. Write down your earliest memories of sex. For example, when and how did you first masturbate? What did you use to get off? What or whom did you fantasize about? What did you feel about your body? Your genitals? Your first time seeing someone else's? Take as long as you need to make this list. Don't rush. Some painful memories, patterns, or trauma may come up in this exercise. I know there have been for me. If it becomes too much, please stop and call a trusted friend or therapist. If you are able to push past some of the things that arise, try to see them as detached from yourself, part of an old system you learned in childhood that no longer serves you.

2. BURN THIS LIST.

3. Now write down all your secret desires. This can include the kind of sex you want to be having, the kind of partnership or love you want to experience, and the relationship you'd like to have with your own body.

4. It's up to you if you want to burn this second list as an intention of what you'd like to draw in or keep it as a reminder as we learn to communicate our desires to close partners.

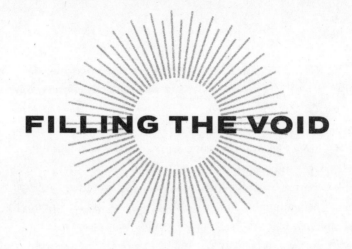

FILLING THE VOID

What needs are we filling when we have sex?

An animal instinct?

A heart connection?

A way to bond with our partner?

A desire to explore our sexuality and pleasure potential?

What about when we choose to enter into a romantic relationship?

Is it because we are deeply in love and feel a soul connection with our partner?

Is it for convenience or financial reasons?

Is it to explore what it means to be truly intimate and seen by another person?

Or do we fear being alone?

Are we settling because it's the best we think we deserve?

Will anyone do?

Do we think that having someone love or desire us means that we are worthy of love?

I f we reach back far enough to our earliest memories, we see that so much of what we have been taught is to link our sense of self-worth and self-esteem to someone else's attention, desire, and love. It feels good to be told as children that we are beautiful, handsome, or good; as awkward teens we want *so badly* to be accepted by our peers, to belong, to be seen as "normal." Through these unconscious experiences, *many of us learned to equate accepting ourselves with having someone else's acceptance.*

Unfortunately, this conditioning leads us to need validation from other people as a way to *love ourselves.* It can cause us to view our desirability, sexuality, and even our worthiness through the lens of whether another person or society as a whole deems us "valuable" or "sexy." Have you ever found yourself wanting someone or something because it would make you feel better about yourself? More complete? "If I only had this job, house, car, partner, sex life, et cetera, then everything would be okay"?

We may find, as adults, that we feel a deep lack—it may even feel like despair—regardless of whether we are in a committed partnership, have our dream job, or are having incredible orgasms all day.

Welcome to *the void.* It is our shadow side and intricately linked to who we are as human beings.

Self-help gurus, "mindfulness" blogs and retreats, detox diets, yoga classes, influencers, and celebrities alike hawk products (hair vitamins! tummy tea!) and ideologies that promise to banish the void and all our dark thoughts in promise of better sex! Happier relationships! A more attractive you!

These are lies.

Any ideal of constant "perfection" and "bliss" is totally unattainable and not all that it's cracked up to be. Some people call trying to suppress or avoid our shadow side "spiritual bypassing." Truth is, we can't experience the great highs without acknowledging and accepting the depths of our lows. Light needs shadow to exist.

More often than not, we think our sex and love lives will fulfill our desire to experience continual happiness, joy, and ecstasy. If only we could stay in a state of perpetual high, we could avoid our void, which can manifest as uncertainty, anxiety, fear, or shame. Name an emotion you'd rather not feel and that, my darling, is your void talking. Sex is a good place to avoid the void. I cannot tell you how many times I am asked to give advice on "how to reach peak orgasm every time."

Here's the reality.

It is impossible to reach your peak every single time. Anyone who promises you that is selling a false bill of goods. If we lived consistently at a peak, we would eventually tire of it. Sometimes an orgasm is stronger than other times; for those with vaginas, sometimes we can only get off with clitoral stimulation, sometimes we can achieve a deep cervical fix. So many factors affect our libido: mood, menstrual cycle, environmental and life stressors, whether or not we are on birth control or antidepressants. When we expect to achieve bliss with every orgasm, we put additional pressure on ourselves instead of being in the moment and experiencing what is actually happening.

It is totally *normal* not to peak, cum, orgasm, ejaculate, squirt, get off with every sexual experience—whether you're doing it with a partner or masturbating. Sometimes you just can't get there physiologically, mentally, or otherwise. Instead of accepting this as a result of being a human and not a robot, we tend to self-flagellate, feel shame, or wonder what is wrong with us.

We have to stop looking at sex as goal or orgasm based. Remember, sex doesn't need to include penetration or an orgasmic outcome. We have to widen our ideas of what a normal sexual experience can be. Not to say a quick fuck with an incredible orgasm isn't what you need sometimes, but you'll only make yourself more frustrated if you expect every encounter to be unicorns and rainbows.

When you notice yourself focusing on a goal during sex, I suggest slowing down, taking some deep breaths, tuning in to your body, and seeing what evolves when you let go of a desired result. We are going to get deep into breath practice later in this book to help us connect with our genitals and achieve improved orgasms.

Experiences and emotions are like waves. We can be riding a high, joyful and ecstatic, or we can feel like we're getting sucked up in the undertow, lonely, insecure, angry, heartbroken, vengeful, bored, anxious, depressed, scared, hurt, self-destructive, sad. Most of us have been taught since childhood to label our undertow emotions as "bad" and the highs as "good" and to ignore, heal, or hide the "bad" emotions as quickly as possible. How many times have you been told not to be sad?

Even if we know that, like a set of waves, our "negative" feelings will eventually pass, it's really hard to sit with them. It might take only a few minutes before we start searching for anything that will distract our brain from the pain we are experiencing. As adults we've reached a point where we are *so good* at disregarding uncomfortable feelings that often we can't even identify the root cause making us want to crawl out of our skin. We will search for anyone or anything to divert our attention from our shadow, our *void*.

Have you ever noticed yourself mindlessly using sex, drugs, food, or alcohol to self-soothe or self-validate? I definitely have. When I was faced with overwhelm, one of my go-to methods for escapist self-soothing was to buy rolling tobacco (I supposedly quit smoking cigarettes at nineteen) to mix with cannabis (which I do appreciate). I'd do this to convince myself that I was smoking a joint instead of just admitting I want to smoke this thing that is "bad" for me, a.k.a. nicotine. But I wouldn't stop there. I'd end up chain-smoking spliff after spliff to get the nicotine fix until my lungs hurt and I felt nauseous. Then I'd throw away the tobacco in a huff . . . only to fish it out of the garbage later and start all over again. The cycle ended only when I either gave the pack of tobacco to a friend (who, thankfully, knows and loves me for my eccentricities) or poured water inside the package and *then* threw it away for good. I *could* just have smoked the cannabis joint and enjoyed the experience, but my trip was to make it into a forbidden overindulgence.

Or maybe you have heard the phrase "eating my feelings"? During the 2016 and 2020 US presidential debates, I could not eat enough chocolate bars to pacify my intense anxiety. I love chocolate, but this was something else: I could go through two or three bars in twenty minutes watching those debates, never mind the stomachache that followed. And then . . . repeat.

This kind of behavior is called *filling a void*. When we mindlessly use [insert your escapism of choice here, whether it be sex, food, drugs, or anything else] to fill a void, we are *avoiding* feeling hard emotions. My chocolate bars were an instant gratification fix that substituted sweets for something I really didn't want to feel (distress over the state of America).

Unfortunately, it can be habit-forming to fill a void through instant gratification, to the point of excess, with things we actually savor. As challenging as it may sound, sometimes we need to pause, witness our discomfort, and process it before proceeding. If we can get quiet enough to notice the feeling we are trying to avoid, we can start to observe it, like a wave. Instead of getting sucked into the undertow, we can watch it crash on the shore and roll out again to sea.

Hard truth: it's not easy to sit in a "bad" feeling without wanting to distract yourself. And sometimes you just need to. But pausing and observing our discomfort, for even a few minutes, helps us understand *why* we are eating chocolate, drinking a martini, smoking a joint, or fucking this person. If we can shift our thinking from *I just really need to fuck because I don't want to feel my heartbreak* to *I am heartbroken, and it sucks, and I just really need to feel validated by another person desiring me*, then we become that much closer to knowing our boundaries and wishes around sex and love.

Our shadow side, or void, is deeply connected to our feelings of self-worth and self-esteem. When we are triggered by something or someone, often we can go so dark and "negative" that we may feel numb, hopeless, or unworthy of sex or love—*even* if we read the self-help books, meditate, pray, and follow all the mindfulness techniques we have learned. *This is normal.* We are *human.* Again, we cannot exist in the light all the time. If we look at religious or spiritual figures throughout history—of all faiths—we will find most of them grappling with the balance of their shadow and light. So when people tell you how perfect their life is or that they have no shadow, you've got to wonder what void they are trying to avoid.

While working on this chapter, I had a conversation with a well-meaning friend who suggested that my previous history of falling for "broken people" could have been easily solved by settling for "a nice, normal person" like her husband, who "has no shadow side." Before we unpack this problematic advice, let me take you to a time when I felt there was nowhere lower I could go. My void, or place of lack, was all I could see.

December 25, 2014. I was in the hospital with my father, who was dying. He had just come out of several days in the intensive care unit, and I knew, intuitively, he just had weeks to live. Christmas Day is also my birthday (a curse as a kid, because everyone forgets your birthday or gives you one gift; now it doesn't bother me). Everyone in my family had gone off on holidays with their partners and kids. Divorced and childless at the time, I made the decision to stay in Los Angeles and be with my dad. I knew how scared he was of dying—he confided this to me the night before he went into the ICU. I thought about how I would feel in my last days, how I couldn't face the idea of not having someone there to comfort me.

Cut to my birthday in the hospital with Dad, me holding his hand and us holding back tears as we watched *It's a Wonderful Life* on the little TV above his bed. He squeezed my hand, turned to me, and said, "I just really want to see you settled, Lizzie." His words struck a deep chord. I wanted so badly to have the same: to feel settled, for him to see me happy in another long-term partnership, for him to know my future child.

In the days that followed, my void overtook me. I longed for anything to stop the self-loathing and lack I felt. Did I choose meditation, prayer, or calling upon one of the many nurturing relationships I have for comfort?

Of course not.

I decided to let the fuckboy[6] who had been trying to bed me for the last eight months visit one night. I definitely didn't tell him my father was dying. As we sat on my couch, did I feel reassured? Did I take my mind off my grief? Nope. He proceeded to dry hump me, finishing by masturbating all over my leg and couch. I chose to turn to a person and experience that made me feel even worse than I already did. And I had no one to blame but myself. Today, I think about this time in my life whenever low self-esteem and self-worth start to overtake me. Alone during the holidays on my birthday with a dying father and dried cum on my couch.

No amount of love or sex will ever fill our void if we don't learn how to love ourselves—and our void.

Especially when it comes to sex, there is so much pressure these days to have mindless, unconnected, and unfulfilling intimacy—from the transactional nature of dating and hook-up apps (no shade, just pointing out the premise of a quick-fix hit of dopamine here) to the dogma shoved down our throats by social media and the greater culture that our value is directly correlated to how sexually attractive we are or how many "likes" our thirst trap receives. The problem is that when we associate sex with a way to escape a feeling we don't want to feel, we also dilute our potential for knowing truly connected (and even transcendent) *pleasure.*

It can be really hard to get to the bottom of what our personal (I'm going to keep drilling it in that *our sexual identity is unique to each of us, like our fingerprints*) motivations are when it comes to sex. We must be able to tune out what works for other people, their advice, and what we see in the media and tune in to what works *for us.* (Remember, our *new normal.*)

It's often said that where thought goes, energy flows.

For me, sometimes a break from being intimate with other people can serve as a healthy opportunity to be more conscious about the sex I have. I've gone through several periods of self-imposed celibacy—immediately postdivorce and after two painful breakups—to reset my heart. My version of celibacy includes masturbation and also kissing and touching someone else, depending on the circumstances and my level of comfort. It could even include spanking and oral sex. What self-imposed celibacy means to me is not being penetrated

---

6   This term generally connotes a male-identified or male-presenting person who remains at the beck and call of those who find them attractive, easily accessing them (usually via text) at a moment's notice for no-strings sexual fulfillment. They often develop a rigid emotional distance, not allowing sexual partners long-term romantic intimacy.

by another person. This allows me to be very clear in my intentions and relationships, to really consider whether I'm using sex to fill a void.

I've found it interesting to observe how often people conflate how much sex you're having with a value judgment on self-worth. How many times has a casual acquaintance asked, "Who are you sleeping with?" or "Who are you seeing?" Have you ever felt ashamed because the answer was "Myself"?

If I had a dollar for every time I've heard a long-coupled (often cis-het[7] and married) person drill a single person about their sex life as though they are trying to live vicariously through them, I would have ten billion dollars. I want to interrupt and ask, "How much sex are you and your spouse having? Do you like anal?" Or even, "What void are you trying to fill by pressuring someone to spill personal details about their sex life? Are you not getting enough at home?" Let this serve as a not-so-gentle reminder that asking people intimate questions about sex without an open "I consent to you digging into my private life" is just inappropriate. Sex Etiquette 101!

But I digress. Getting back to my occasional practice of self-imposed celibacy, the more open I've been about taking these periods for myself, the more I've heard from others that they are having a lot less sex than they let on—regardless of relationship status.

When I say the word *celibacy*, what do you picture? A monk taking a vow of chastity? Someone denying themselves pleasure? Do you think of incels posting misogynistic threads to Reddit in the dark? Do you imagine someone saving themselves for marriage or God? Do you think that if you go too long without penetrative sex, your genitals will grow cobwebs? Do you consider celibacy the absence of all orgasms—including via masturbation? Have you ever gone through a period of self-imposed celibacy?

Professionally through The Sex Ed and personally, I want to encourage people to be open and accepting of other people's choices, whether that means polyamory, sex parties, fetishes, or the decision to take a break.

Here are excerpts from some conversations on celibacy with friends and colleagues. They've enlightened my perspective and made me feel less isolated

---

7   *Cis-het* is slang shorthand for "cisgender heterosexual," *cisgender* meaning someone who identifies with the gender assigned to them at birth by the medical community. The term can apply to those of any and all sexual orientations, meaning that a cisgender woman can identify as heterosexual, homosexual, bisexual, or any of the endlessly evolving definitions of sexual attraction. *Heterosexual* means someone who subscribes to a male-female definition of relationships or marriage.

when I've gone through periods focused on *self-love*. We also talked about whether, when having sex with a partner, we are using them or the act itself just to *fill a void.*

My friend Gila Shlomi, also known as "Weezy," is a sexpert and cohost of the *WHOREible Decisions* podcast, devoted to breaking down the kinky-sex stigmas for people of color. She is open to all kinds of new experiences, from being dragged (by me) to a kundalini class to attending a Zoom orgy . . . and then some. Despite her adventuresomeness, she shared with me that

> through certain breakups I need to be celibate until I feel like I'm over this moment. Because [if I don't,] then I'm just going to be having sex to cover the pain up. We think that sex is going to solve those feelings or make us feel better, which it doesn't. I think that when we think of someone being totally celibate, we have this image of a nun who can't do anything. That's what I kind of had to learn: "Oh, I can be sexy and sexual but not have sex." People don't look at celibacy as a journey into discovering yourself more than they do a pity party.

Carolyn Murphy is a supermodel who has graced the covers of American, French, and Italian *Vogue*, was the face of the longest running cosmetic campaign in the business (for Estée Lauder), and walks runways all over the world. You'd think someone who is canonized for her beauty and desirability would have just as enviable a sex life, right? But according to Carolyn,

> I've been celibate in between the majority of my relationships. I think the maximum time I've gone was five years of not having sex. And I didn't have any contact with a man, not even a kiss. Sometimes [when people find out I've been celibate] you get the wide eyes, like, "Oh my God, how could you do that?" I'm not at a loss for finding somebody to have sex with. This is something that I'm choosing. I just have a lot of other ways that I'm fulfilling myself right now. I think that's usually the shocker for people. I've had girlfriends be like, "You've got to get that shit moving. You've got to get going." And I'm like, "No, I'm not giving up this golden pussy for just anybody, that shit's sacred." Somebody's got to earn getting into that.

More women spoke openly to me about celibacy than men, perhaps because masculine identity has been very much tied up with the idea of sexual prowess, making it more shameful or "abnormal" (there we go again with that "normal" holding us back!) for men to admit *choosing* not to partake. However, even highly successful men who could have their pick of partners have chosen periods of celibacy.

Ramy Youssef, comedian, director, and writer, is the Golden Globe–winning creator and star of *Ramy* on Hulu. His show explores many themes surrounding sex—from faith to filling the void—as his character tries to find the middle ground between earthly desires and the divine. One episode opens with him in bed, furiously eating Haribo gummies and masturbating to porn. Ultimately, both make him feel sick. **"I didn't want to have sex until I got married, and so I didn't until my early twenties,"** he said. **"It was the thing that was happening in high school, very much so, but for me, I didn't want to, and then I took an acting class and that messed everything up. You're in acting class and you're like, 'Oh, man. I've got to express myself.'"** Even after becoming sexually active, he still chose to go through periods of celibacy to get a better understanding of his relationship to and boundaries around sex and faith. **"It's just to be able to pause. I think dudes, we have a really hard time pausing. We're always just like, 'Wait, I did what?' A dude before sex and after sex is like a time machine. He's like, 'Oh, man. I'm different.' It can really be an intoxicating experience, I think."**

I've known musician, producer, and mad musical scientist Mark Ramos Nishita for more than two decades. In addition to his solo work, "Money Mark" has collaborated with the Beastie Boys, the Talking Heads' David Byrne, and the Yeah Yeah Yeahs, among many others. He admitted, **"There's been countless times, I mean dozens and dozens of times, where I would rather masturbate than have sex with a person. Early when I was growing up, I would just have sex with someone if they wanted to have sex. And then later I felt like, *What am I doing if I'm not really connecting with this person?* It was kind of empty sex, is that what they call it? I just felt that there wasn't any, like, value to it, and I would just rather masturbate and call it a day."**

It's not just civilians I spoke with who noticed they were using sex to fill a void; even some of the biggest names in the adult industry, who are literally *paid* to have sex, find comfort in abstaining. Joanna Angel is a multiple-award-winning adult film star, director, producer, author, entrepreneur, and founder of the alt-porn adult studio Burning Angel Entertainment, which she launched in

2002—while in college. "There was a while when I didn't count my on-camera sex as getting laid," she revealed. "When I was in between one relationship and another, I went a good amount of time without off-camera sex. I know nobody will feel bad for me. I was still having really good on-camera sex. To me that was celibacy." She also went through a celibate period before she started working in porn:

> I was in a relationship and was so sad when it ended. The guy
> cheated on me, and I was devastated, heartbroken. I remember
> trying to cope with it by having a whole bunch of sloppy, drunken,
> desperate-feeling one-night stands. The sex wasn't coming from a
> good place. I was like, *All right, I'm just going to stop thinking about
> sex.* I masturbated. Masturbating is really good for you. People forget
> when they really feel the need to get laid, that need can go away by
> just taking care of yourself. Take the edge off, so then when you go
> out there in the world and you're ready to meet someone, you can
> give them the best version of you and not this desperate, anxious,
> on-edge version of you. I want sex to be fun and a beautiful moment
> that you're sharing with someone, not something that is almost like
> an addiction you need to fill.

If masturbation is self-love, it may be one of the healthiest ways to fill the void. Here's a new mantra to remember if you find yourself getting really dark. Before you reach for whatever/whoever is your go-to void filler: *meditate, music, masturbate.* Meaning, take a beat before you eat/fuck/get high/ drink and notice whether you are doing it for pleasure or to escape. For me, this means meditating (which might be twenty minutes of sitting quietly or a quick cleansing breath work that I will cover later in this book); playing music I love to dance or sing along to (my friend Grace Harry suggested I make a happy songs playlist); followed by some self-soothing action, a.k.a. getting myself off! If the urge is still there (but often it isn't after the above), then I'll indulge.

So how do we learn to live with our voids? Here are some helpful steps to remember when the shadow self peers from our darkest recesses:

1. Acknowledge and love your shadow. It is part of you, and the more you reject it (reject *you*) the harder it (*you*) will be to escape.

2. Try to sit with uncomfortable emotions long enough to realize where they are coming from. If the *meditate, music, masturbate* mantra above doesn't work for you, here is a simple practice. Set a timer for two minutes. Close your eyes and tune in to the feeling you are trying to avoid. Is it fear, loneliness, a lack of self-worth? Anxiety? Boredom? Where do you feel it in your body? Is your chest tight? Your stomach clenched? When the timer goes off, freewrite for another two minutes about where you think these feelings are coming from. Just taking a pause (if you have kids, think of it as giving yourself a time-out) can help you establish whether it is you or your void running the show.

3. Get cozy with your void. Sometimes we just feel empty, and that is okay. To be human is to live in a gray area. Everything doesn't have to look or feel perfect.

So I'll ask you again the questions I did at the start of this chapter:

> What needs are we are filling when we have sex?
> An animal instinct?
> A heart connection?
> A way to bond with our partner?
> A desire to explore our sexuality and pleasure potential?
> What about when we choose to enter into a romantic relationship?
> Is it because we are deeply in love and feel a soul connection with our partner?
> Is it for convenience or financial reasons?
> Is it to explore what it means to be truly intimate and seen by another person?
> Or do we fear being alone?
> Are we settling because it's the best we think we deserve?
> Will anyone do?
> Do we think that having someone love or desire us means that we are worthy of love?

Knowing our motivations helps us keep clear in our sexual relationships: What are we fulfilling or what are we trying to avoid feeling?

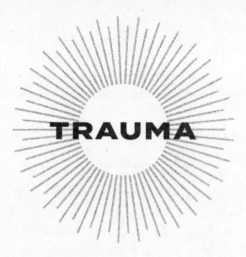

TRAUMA

Before we begin, let me emphasize that I am not an expert in trauma therapy, and I encourage people to seek professional support. This is a really tender topic, and no one should have to go through processing alone or before they are ready. The following stories, tools, and practices have helped me begin to work through and communicate my own traumas. I share them in the hopes that they might offer solace to others with similar experiences. Wherever possible, I have noted qualified and licensed experts who specialize in these issues and what to look for (and ask up front) when you are seeking counsel.

Unprocessed trauma is one of our biggest barriers to pleasure. What traumas must we acknowledge and communicate in order to have healthier, more loving and sexual relationships with ourselves and our partners?

Most humans have been through some kind of trauma. When we think of trauma, we normally associate it with distressing experiences or physical injuries. These can include sexual assault, death of a loved one, divorce, abortion, miscarriage, family fissure, hate crimes, domestic violence, mental illness, alcoholism or drug addiction (yours or a loved one's), incarceration, living in an environment where you are experiencing high stress due to climate disaster, a pandemic, or political instability.

Traumas can also include what may, on the surface, seem minor, such as microaggressions, which build up over time; a car accident or sports injury; a personal or career loss. Just because something *appears* less than tragic does not make it any less impactful to your emotional and sexual well-being. We recently received an email to our site from a young woman who was distressed that every time she orgasmed she burst into tears. She was even further troubled that she couldn't name what she considered a singular massive traumatic event to attribute this to, such as an assault. Point being, the way our bodies and psyches react to trauma is, like our sexual identities, highly dependent on our individual experiences.

Trauma is not comfortable to think about, let alone discuss aloud. Our thoughts may be consumed with heavy tragedy and loss, yet we answer "How are you?" with "I'm fine" because it's easier than telling the truth. And we all are so well trained in avoiding the awkward truth, right? Even though we are all secretly experiencing the same difficult process of moving through life, ahh . . . we humans are so good at conforming to the norm . . . sigh.

Here is the truth: *Our trauma makes us uncomfortable. Other people's trauma makes us uncomfortable.*

We tend to sweep under the rug complex topics like sex, death, and grief. Yet the less we talk about the deep sadness and traumas that we all share as humans, the more power we give them over us.

Here's where our old friend the void comes in. When we start to face our void, instead of ignoring or filling it, trauma tends to resurface—sometimes for the first time—exhibiting itself as a dull ache or a sharp pain. Other times it can manifest as a huge, knock-you-down, can't-get-up, never-even-knew-it-was-there-to-begin-with emotional event.

Although on a personal level we may want (or be well trained anthropologically) to avoid feeling, naming, or honoring our trauma, culturally we are inundated with images of trauma on every front, from violence and disaster-related plotlines in blockbuster movies to the mass death, disaster, and bloodshed we bear witness to globally. Adding to that, much of the sexual material we consume as entertainment or news centers around "trauma porn." This includes the barrage of sexual violence depicted in our favorite streaming shows and the countless cases of sexual assault and harrassment that fill our daily social media feeds.

There's a disconnect between our inability to recognize or reconcile our personal traumas while having trauma shoved down our throats the second we look at our devices. Is this our sick trick of confronting trauma in a "safe" way—so we don't have to deal with our own? Is it easier to cry and break down about things happening outside of ourselves than to face the darkness we experience firsthand? At the height of the 2020 COVID-19 lockdowns, most of the world was glued to the news, watching our collective trauma unfold, sharing death rates and apocalyptic articles—often instead of sharing our uncertainty and fear with one another.

Especially when it comes to sex, most of what we see in mainstream culture unfortunately is linked to trauma. Most entertainment, news reports, and even educational discussion around sex, particularly in the past ten years, focuses on assault, consent, or methods to avoid pregnancy and STIs.

Where is our healthy modeling around *pleasure* when it comes to sex? Where, outside of pornography, can we witness sensual, consensual, and joyous celebrations of sexuality? Where is the space we are carving out to experience the consciousness-expanding possibilities of sex? Where are we seeing that sex and our sexuality are key to becoming the most fulfilled versions of ourselves we can possibly be?

Perhaps this is a reflection of where we are as a society and how much we have kept our traumas from the light. But the light is where we can find community, support, and acceptance for some of our most vulnerable experiences.

There is also one type of trauma we all share some form of, beyond our individual stories: ancestral.

The stories, patterns, and traumas of our parents, grandparents, and other forebears (even if we are unaware of them) get passed down to us. Ancestral trauma is intertwined with racial, gender, and sexual systems that have long confined, defined, and oppressed us. Those with ancestors who were born or forced into slavery; indigenous people whose land was taken from them; those whose languages were stripped away, who have suffered centuries of racial attacks and other injustices—all carry trauma inside their DNA. On the opposite end of the spectrum of oppression is the ancestral trauma of those whose ancestors exploited, abused, and/or owned enslaved people. There must be acknowledgment of both the scars we carry and the sins of our lineage in order for healing to take place.

Many of us also carry trauma around sexual abuse and assault that we and our friends, mothers, grandmothers, great-grandmothers, great-great-grandmothers, and so on up the line have suffered for centuries. I'm speaking about the collective matriarchal line here. Though not all survivors of assault have vaginas, historically it has been more prevalent. The premise many cultures have been built on is that the victor, as a righteous spoil of war, has the right to rape and capture women of the village as due rewards.

On our patriarchal line, we have another type of trauma to contend with: a cycle of behavior that rewards conquest, pillage, violence, abuse, and what some call "toxic" but I prefer to call "wounded" masculinity. This line doesn't encourage weakness or sensitivity (in fact, it actively discourages these yin[8] traits). I imagine it must be suffocating to have all these projections placed upon what it is to be "masculine."

Just as women have experienced thousands of years of violence and oppression, so too have men been locked in boxes by the patriarchal framework of our culture; kept from experiencing nurturing, soft, and vulnerable spaces as containers to help them heal from traumatic events; and been told to "suck it up" and "be a man." I wonder how many buried traumas have been expressed as anger, violence, sexual frustration, and assault.

As I write this chapter, I know I can call upon a vast support network, both in real life and virtually, to help process the trauma that is coming up from plumbing these depths. There is so much more community than ever before for women, nonbinary, and LBGTQIA+[9] folks to openly share and normalize our wounds. But where do these places exist for heterosexual men? Where and how do we provide support and encouragement to heterosexual men so they can heal their own deep, dark spaces of hurt? Do we expect heterosexual men to evolve with the times we are in, yet leave them on their own to find assistance and community?

Prior to the 1990s (riot grrrl, Anita Hill hearings, post–feminist wave), sexual assault was *not discussed* privately or publicly. There were no openly promoted support groups or health services for survivors. I helped start a rape and sexual assault support group in my own progressive, sex-positive high school in the midnineties. My school was among the first in America to pass out condoms to students to promote safe sex and have an LGBTQIA+ history class—yet talking about sexual trauma was still embarrassing and taboo. I remember being angry back then that there were

---

8   Yin and yang: This concept of dualism and balance (yin being the receptive principle, and yang being the active) originated in ancient Chinese philosophy. Its symbolization of mutually dependent binary forces can be applied to a variety of contexts, ranging from conventional assessments of sex (dominant, submissive), gender (male, female), and sexuality (penetrative, receptive) to more esoteric considerations of group psychology and even of shadow and light. It centers the notions of balance, equity, and reciprocity in these contexts, fundamentally noting each person's capacity to exhibit both sides of any coin and the importance of the interconnectedness of both sides—for instance, the idea that not only do dark and light coexist but the dark needs the light and vice versa, bringing us to the phrase's translation of "dark and bright."

9   These letters represent those who identify as lesbian, gay, bisexual, transgender, queer, intersex, and asexual. The plus sign indicates commitment to the term's range of identities broadening indefinitely.

no real justice system penalties in place for abuse. (This still is an area where we are sorely lacking.) Survivors of abuse were disowned and/or shamed by their family, society, and even themselves. Imagine no cultural access to therapy or healing. At all. Imagine how many incidents of untreated assault over the years this amounts to. All this pain and trauma hidden in the proverbial closet, left to breed fear, shame, rage, depression, panic, lack of desire, excessive sexual proclivities, deep sadness. Many survivors describe a feeling of being broken.

When we come into the world, regardless of whether we have a personal experience of assault, we already carry these ancestral traumas in our genes. If you trace your genealogy back far enough (and you may be surprised or heartbroken to see that you don't need to go too far), you will discover many stories of sexual trauma in your own family whether it be about your mother, grandma, aunt, sister, uncle, brother, or cousin.

Maybe they shared the story of their abuse with you when you were a kid, and you didn't know how to process it. Many kids who witness or learn that a close family member was violated absorb that feeling and spend years thinking the abuse happened to them. Maybe you didn't believe the stories you heard or resented them or judged them. Or maybe you are a survivor yourself.

For many years after my mother shared her story with me of being sexually molested as a child, I had a visceral reaction, as though I had experienced the assault myself. I remember feeling sick to my stomach and clenching my vagina as she related her experience. Even now, as I think about those I love who have or are suffering abuse, or when I look back on the times in which my own sexual boundaries were violated, it takes me to a place where the thought of being "sexy" is the last thing on my mind. My body goes into a state of panic and threat, even if I am with a supportive partner.

Though we now have more systems and support in place to process sexual trauma than we have in the past, we still have an expectation that there will be a resolution eventually, that one day it'll just go away and you/they will be "healed." Even if we, our partner, our friend, or a family member has dealt extensively with processing their trauma, there may still be things that trigger us. You could be in the middle of a sexual act you enjoy and have participated in with full enthusiastic consent hundreds of times with someone you love and old wounds may resurface. *This is normal. You are okay.*

If this happens, stop any sexual activity, regroup, and tell your partner that you feel triggered. Ask for what you need to feel safe. Anyone who is lucky enough to be intimate with you should always respect your sexual boundaries, as you would theirs. If you or your partner are working through personal trauma, having ongoing, continuously renewed sexual consent is especially important as you uncover these layers.

Any kind of trauma—no matter whether major or minor—has the capacity to shake our foundational core and impact our ability to *be in our bodies*, feel sexual, experience pleasure, and truly let ourselves go with a partner.

Even if we have spent time and energy and have done therapy to deal with our traumas and PTSD, there is no point in which these experiences are not *part of us*. Unfortunately, we cannot control when our traumas or pain rears its head: we can literally be brought to our knees by a sound, fluctuating hormones, a color, a touch, a smell, or a change in the season. Strong emotions and sex can also bring deep reservoirs of pain flooding back. I was in a new relationship shortly after my father died, and the sex was amazing—yet right in the midst of waves of intense multiple orgasms I started sobbing uncontrollably. My orgasm had opened a floodgate of emotions. I looked down at the end of the bed, and my cat was biting my lover's feet while I came, which suddenly turned my tears into hysterical laughter. Sex and intimacy can induce such heightened states that control over our reactions goes out the window. Much like the young woman who wrote in for advice about her crying orgasms, at the time my conscious mind didn't connect the incident with grief or past trauma. It was only in retrospect that I put together the pieces.

As we move through life, at some point, most of us will experience trauma. Whether we bury it or face it directly, it may feel like we will never move through it, that we won't ever be "complete" or "healed." Trauma may make us feel so deeply ashamed that we think no one else could ever love us or see us as anything but "damaged goods." In fact, our traumas, while painful, are just another part of the individual stories (and scars) that *make us who we are*. Yes, experiencing trauma can cause extreme vulnerability; but this vulnerability may become more of an asset than a liability to our growth and to deepening our intimate relationships. Revealing our insecurities, "flaws," and complicated personal histories allows us to be *seen*. We fall in love with others (and they fall in love with us) when we are able to witness and reveal vulnerability as well as our deepest hurt. Of course, this is not going to happen overnight! It takes time and trust to reveal ourselves. This is why we need to be wary of love bombing,[10] particularly if we have a history of trauma, as we may be especially vulnerable to over-the-top and immediate declarations of love. Going slow allows us to notice our feelings instead of getting lost in the fix/save/heal-my-wounds sauce.

The Japanese have a beautiful aesthetic called *wabi sabi* that celebrates imperfection, impermanence, and incompleteness. A technique called *kintsugi* is used to fill in the cracks of a piece of broken ceramic with gold. It is also applied as a philosophy to let go of an attachment to perfection or wholeness. It is the cracks themselves that are to be adored.

Could we possibly find a way to love our trauma or at least that part of ourselves that we may see as damaged? If there are literal scars on our bodies—for example, postpartum—can we consider a practice of loving and even worshipping these scars as symbolic of our strength? Whether you undergo an easy vaginal birth, a complicated labor, or a scheduled C-section, every birth adventure exacts some kind of physical and emotional toll. Can we be tender to ourselves and reframe the stitches and marks on our bodies in a loving way? For new mothers healing from labor who have little desire or physical wherewithal to engage in penetration, it can be empowering to simply spend some time caretaking your vulva. This can include gently applying lubrication or holding a mirror to yourself to get acquainted with the changes your glorious body has just been through. I know it is easier to self-flagellate in front of the mirror rather than compliment ourselves, but it is good to get in the practice of self-validation rather than seeking outside acceptance. When we can see beauty within our pain, it becomes easier to love and embrace ourselves, scars, trauma, and all.

Hawaiian culture gives some insight into how we can honor trauma. Lei Wann, director of Limahuli Garden and Preserve on the island of Kauai, broke down for me how one of the essential Hawaiian creation myths plus a diet staple, the taro (or *kalo*) plant, help people integrate the loss of a child:

---

10 This term describes the act of lavishing attention in the form of gifts, grand gestures, persistence, flattery, and constant contact early in a relationship with the narcissistic goal of gaining power and control over the recipient. It can be an insidious form of emotional abuse, with potential for escalating into future abuse. Love bombing is further complicated by the fact that it's been celebrated in romantic literature and films for years. Many now are reconsidering their previous affection for knights in shining armor and Prince Charmings like Edward Cullen, Noah Calhoun, and Christian Gray.

According to Hawaiian mythology, Wakea (the sky father) and the beautiful goddess Ho'ohokukalani (the heavenly one who made the stars) wished to have a child. Their first attempt resulted in a stillbirth. The body of the stillborn child was buried near their home. From this grew a taro (kalo) plant; the plant was named Haloanaka (long stock trembling). The couple's second attempt at a child resulted in a human boy, which the gods named Haloa. Hawaiian families will name and honor their miscarriages and often bury them on the eastern corner of their house. If you ask someone how many children they have, they will include any children they have lost to stillbirth.

This way of *living* with trauma allows for grief, anger, and all the other challenging emotions associated with loss to be part of the natural cycle.

Might we hold this quality of space for the trauma of an abortion? Whether or not to have an abortion is a tough decision no matter where you stand on reproductive rights. We have so much support for those experiencing childbirth but little open dialogue on aftercare when it comes to choosing to terminate a pregnancy. Can we imagine honoring an abortion with a ceremony of acceptance and release for the trauma we have experienced in our wombs? My friend Erica Chidi is a doula, author, and cofounder of LOOM, an educational reproductive-health resource platform. She points out that

there are doulas that work with people through miscarriages, abortions, or stillbirths. All of those experiences are reproducti[on] related. A lot of the same physiology is happening on a continuum through all those experiences. People need emotional and educational support, regardless of what the outcome looks like. Getting an abortion for a lot of people is health-seeking behavior. You are not wanting to be pregnant because of a myriad of reasons. If we start to look at it as health-seeking behavior, then it makes sense that there needs to be doula support. Just being there, holding space for them as they're dealing with all of these uncomfortable physiological sensations. And the emotional sensations that are really challenging as well. Everybody deserves really good, evidence-based, nonjudgmental emotional support for big life changes.

Just as our muscles spasm during a car accident or sports injury, our womb may be a primary place of holding trauma and tension, whether it be from pregnancy, miscarriage, stillbirth, abortion, vaginismus, assault— or even from a nonreproductive, nonsexually related incident. There are pelvic floor therapists all around the world who specialize in a massage technique known as pelvic floor massage, which focuses on the pelvic floor muscles, connective tissues, and ligaments. You can also practice pelvic floor massage on yourself, after consulting with a medical advisor and trying it with a licensed professional.

When you work with a pelvic floor therapist, the internally based massage should be preceded by an intake session in which the practitioner explains all aspects of the treatment and you sign an informed consent form. This means you have a clear understanding of the type of massage work that will take place, which may include clean, gloved hands being inserted into the perineum and/ or vulva for the purpose of muscle release.

Even as an avid devotee of bodywork, I hadn't realized how essential it was to address my own reproductive organs as part of my overall physical and emotional wellness until I experienced a pelvic floor massage firsthand. And this was after referring people out to specialists for years! Sure, it may be a little intimidating at first to consider a total stranger massaging your vulva, uterus, or perineum, but it's more akin to visiting a doctor with very good bedside manners. (Let me be clear that this is not sexual and, as mentioned above, involves clear discussion around boundaries and consent beforehand.)

In a typical gynecological exam, the gloved hand of your physician is inside you for less than five minutes, to check for irregularities and perform a Pap smear. During a pelvic floor massage, you have a longer opportunity to connect to your internal and reproductive organs and to do so in a way you may never have experienced. It is normal for trauma to come up, for tears to be shed, and even for tight muscles to deeply relax.

During my session, my therapist was communicating with me, making sure I was comfortable, asking what was coming up for me, and explaining where she was going to massage next. I found it fascinating to notice that, for example, my G-spot was tight internally. When she was working on my right ovary, I had intense anxiety and flashed back to being eight years old, when my mother told me about her molestation. All these years later, and I was still holding on to that memory in my womb. My therapist told me that some people she works with may have months of sessions that involve just talking, no touch. Others may need multiple sessions of massage or come in only once for an overall tune-up.

The thing about trauma is that it is way too overwhelming for our minds to handle or process all at once. Let's take the COVID-19 pandemic, for example. Globally, we experienced such mass loss, grief, financial and emotional instability, isolation, and mental stress that it will be years before we can really understand and heal from our collective PTSD. And for many around the world, the trauma of the COVID pandemic triggered flashbacks to previous personal wounds and suffering. This is normal and can happen if you experience any kind of trauma. In his seminal book *Waking the Tiger: Healing Trauma*, psychotherapist Peter Levine wrote that "to confront trauma head on, it will continue to do what it has already done—immobilize us in fear." Even a minor car accident can uncover feelings of grief from something that you'd locked away and hoped never to feel again. Again, we simply cannot control when our trauma decides it's time to deal. It can take years for trauma to resurface, for the mind and body to bear witness.

When I got sick with COVID-19 in February 2020, early in the pandemic, for some reason it brought back memories of living with my ex-husband a couple of blocks from the World Trade Center on 9/11. For almost twenty years I had pushed the sounds and visions of that day away. I never spoke of it, even when among a group of friends talking about where they had been when the Twin Towers fell.

Isolated with COVID, for the first time I had feverish nightmares and lucid dreams of that day. Visions I never wanted to relive. They came in fragments, like short news clips, except I had seen firsthand the burning building, the people jumping out of windows, and I had been covered in ash from head to toe after our windows blew in when the first tower fell. The shock and horror of that day and those to follow were so overwhelming that I had to shut down completely to function. I couldn't watch any news footage; I had panic attacks in underground subways and parking lots; and I experienced severe anxiety. For years I took multiple antianxiety pills when flying to quell the sound of the jet engine. To this day I mentally plot the exit routes in any crowd, concert, or movie theater.

It took almost twenty years for my brain to decide it was time to confront the trauma directly.

It is interesting to think about how animals behave when they are attacked in the wild; they don't respond with the same fight-or-flight response[11] that humans do. You may have seen your pet seeking shelter when there is a lightning storm or their hair stand up on end when in fear mode. Under threat, many animals exhibit a biological response of shaking off the trauma in order to reset their nervous system to a state of well-being. This means they are not still thinking or growling about the attack when they get back to their pack or hive.

When the human nervous system perceives it is under attack—that is, when we undergo trauma, abuse, a car accident, an injury, surgery, a major disaster, or the like—we tense up, grin and bear it, or bury it. The trauma is stored in our body memory and, no matter how much we intellectually process it through talk therapy, our biological reactions don't allow us to forget. Our muscle memory can be so deep and layered that even the thought of having a relaxing massage can cause a panic attack.

Activist and journalist Ashlee Marie Preston is the first openly trans person to run for state office in California, as well as the first trans person to become editor in chief of a nationwide publication. She told me,

> There is so much trauma that I am still holding in my body. I recently had my first massage, and I did not like it. It was super tense. When people say, "Loosen up," I actually feel tense. It's just my default. I'm still learning what pleasure is. For me, as a former survival sex worker, pleasure was literally just a feeling. I can't get out of my head because there's so much stuff. . . . Survivors of rape, which I have been raped in my adult life, we disassociate. In fact, the way that I move throughout the world, probably the reason why I'm able to do everything that I'm doing [professionally], is because I'm not even listening to my body. I'm not even aware [that] I'm not in and I'm just out. [I want to] feel safe enough to return to my own body.

---

11 Coined by psychologist Walter Cannon in the 1920s, this term refers to the instinctive reactions that occur in humans (and animals) during moments of heightened stress or danger. The body's amplified release of hormones often results in an individual instantly either preparing to stay and combat an assailant or flee for safety. Freeze is another common yet lesser-known response. Where fight-or-flight responses enlist the (stimulating) sympathetic nervous system, the freeze response enlists the (calming) parasympathetic nervous system. This means that when the sympathetic nervous system has been stimulated to such a degree that the body can no longer react, the parasympathetic nervous system then seeks to protect the mind and body by shutting down or freezing—more specifically, by doing nothing.

Some people may need to move very slowly into any kind of touch or intimacy, whether in a professional or a romantic situation, in order to honor their trauma. Others may benefit greatly from physical touch as a way to release stored trauma that talk therapy can't access. Our relationship to trauma and how we can process it will vary from person to person. Again, there is no "correct" way to do this. If you find yourself feeling tense in an intimate encounter, it can be helpful to pause and try to identify where the tension is emanating from in your body.

A simple grounding technique that many therapists use and that I have found helpful when in a panic state is to sit in a chair with both feet on the floor. I focus my attention on feeling the four corners of each foot on the ground, my body supported by the chair. The simple act of noticing your body connecting with the object you are sitting on and with the floor itself takes the mind out of the hamster wheel. Another exercise that can be done in any position or with any ability is to notice three things in your environment and name them aloud. For example, if I look up right now from my laptop, in my peripheral vision I see a black spinning fan, a purple orchid, and a pink water bottle. I can keep looking at those three objects or name more. This helps me orient myself into the present moment (right here, right now) instead of my mind taking me to the past or the future. During either of these exercises, the more long, deep breaths you can take, the better. Moving your consciousness from an often wildly spinning inner state into your outer horizon—which can be, quite literally, a spot in the distance or the water stain on your ceiling—can bring you into an actual field of awareness.

Wendy Cherry is a sex therapist and executive director and cofounder of the American Association of Couples and Sex Therapists, or AACAST. Dr. Cherry is also codirector, coordinator, and lecturer for UCLA's AACAST programming, which is directed toward medical residents and undergrads as well as licensed and practicing sex therapists. As I mentioned in the introduction, I met Wendy in 2012 when I began auditing a sex education, therapy, and behavior seminar at UCLA, and she and I became fast friends. She was the first colleague to turn me on to the principles of somatic therapy, which is a type of therapy that integrates mind, body, and spirit, treating the effects of mental and emotional issues, PTSD, and trauma through a body-centric approach as well as talk therapy. This form of therapy can include licensed somatic psychological work as well as massage, energy healing, Reiki, pelvic floor healing, and body movement. "The body holds memories" of trauma," Wendy says:

Unfortunately, unlike animals, most of the time we're not allowed that period of time to get up and shake it off. We are not allowed natural metabolization of trauma. Or we have some notion of judgment around it. I actually have prescribed a mindful massage for patients. With an extremely dismissive type A, can't relax, difficulty connecting, I say, "I want you to go get a massage." Sometimes they will be like, "I've had a massage before." And I say, "No. I want you to focus on one second at a time. Where you're being touched, what your skin is doing under the touch, and just really focus on that for the entire massage." And it's been transformative in some cases. The fact of the matter is, touch is one of the most healing things one human being can do for another. And that's why it's so effective in trauma treatment.

I talked earlier about pelvic floor massage, which is a form of somatic therapy. You may have heard of sex therapy, which is primarily talk based. There are some other somatic therapeutic practices—perhaps less known and understood outside of the sex field—that deal with sexually related issues and involve physical touch, talk therapy, and boundary work. Here, licensed practitioners specialize in creating a consensual, boundaried container for fantasy, pleasure, personal exploration, and healing. Two of the most common types of therapists in this arena, for the purposes outlined in this chapter, are sexological bodyworkers and sex surrogates.

A sexological bodyworker may also be referred to as an intimacy or sex coach. They often utilize a number of modalities, including touch, breath work, pelvic floor and scar tissue release, and erotic massage. My friend, the sexpert and "Glamazon" Tyomi Morgan, is an American College of Sexologists–certified sexologist, a writer, and an "international pleasure coach" with a strong intent to represent people of color within mainstream sexuality. As part of Tyomi's practice, she offers various forms of sexological bodywork. I asked her about her intake process with new clients. Her response should give you an idea of how much communication and consent are involved before any one-on-one work takes place:

I have predetermined questions to get a background on people who come to me for coaching. If they can answer those questions, I'll follow up with more questions to receive more clarity and qualify if we are a good fit to work together. If we are a good fit, I send another intake form that goes more in depth into their sexual history, their health history, family history, and so on. I make it very clear in the contracts I send over what my boundaries are.

When I'm doing in-person coaching, I always let my clients know, especially when it is mostly talk based, that there will be no sexual interaction between us. If we are doing something that is hands-on, I'm always going to get consent and establish consent throughout the entire experience. Most of the time, if it's hands-on, I'm not touching them naked. When it comes to sexological bodywork, a lot of times I do work where myself and the client may be nude, and I'm very explicit about my boundaries during the session. There is no penetrative sex happening, whether that's anal, vaginal, or oral. When it comes to touching me, because we are body to body and close, I always let them know that touching is okay once I give consent for it to be okay. I always leave the door open for clients to ask questions or to raise concerns about things within the coaching that they may feel uncomfortable with or have some difficulty with.

Sex surrogacy is another somatic practice that may or may not include sex (remember sex does not necessarily mean penetration). Sessions are based on the client's needs—or clients', plural, as sex surrogates often work with couples. The client may learn flirting, nonsexual touch, or self-pleasure, as well as sexual skills. Sex surrogacy can be particularly useful with physically or emotionally disabled clients who may need the extra patience and support available in a professional setting to gain sexual experience and skills.

Any worth-your-money-and-time professional sex therapist, surrogate, pelvic floor therapist, or sexological bodyworker should be trauma informed. I would recommend scheduling a virtual consultation before engaging in any real-life touch-based session. It is imperative for the practitioner to be clear about the boundaries of the work and for you to be able to address any concerns or questions you may have. If they are ambiguous as to the nature of the session or you have an "off" feeling, don't engage further. We are going to cover boundaries extensively in the next chapter and how to honor our "off" or gut feelings later on in this book. Either way, you *must feel safe* to work with a professional when it comes to any kind of trauma work around sex.

In situations where we experience intense trauma, it is very common to trauma bond—particularly in a romantic relationship, and especially so in those that are rooted in physical, verbal, emotional, and sexual abuse. Shared suffering, even if you are the one being victimized, creates a powerful attachment that can feel impossible to break. However, within the container of a healthy intimate relationship, trusting someone enough to share our trauma (and having someone trust us enough to be able to share theirs) is a true act of vulnerability. This is not only a beautiful and intimate gift but a great strength.

As much as we may fear the darkness of trauma, the more we avoid it, the more we are held back by it. Yet, as I mentioned before, each of us is on our own schedule when it comes to this odyssey. There's no reason to push against an insurmountable force before you—your body or psyche—are ready.

Trauma can be kind of like that box of photos you can't bring yourself to throw away, yet looking at them triggers feelings you'd rather not experience to pierce every pore of your heart. For example, what box do you put failed long-term relationships or marriages into? What do you do with a box of wedding photos that will never make their way into an album or be on display again? Do you keep them securely hidden in the back of a closet? Burn them? Pull them out when you're eighty? Asking for a friend (a.k.a. myself). I personally like to look at photos of loved ones I've lost to remind myself of good times, while some memories (and people) sit in the shadowy recesses of my mind, collecting dust.

Trauma doesn't just go away; it stays in our cells. It rises when it is ready for our brains to face and integrate it. Often, the more I have resisted feeling the pain again and shoved it down, the more it has pulled at me until I've no choice but to notice it. What I can do now is arm myself with tools to support this process when it comes. For me, this is an ongoing practice, like peeling away layers of an onion—and each layer can make me cry! Then I need to stop and allow myself time to process. Time tells me when I am able to go deeper. Many of the things I am working through are taking years to face. My tools have included talk therapy, somatic therapy (massage, pelvic floor work, movement exercises), and learning how to recognize when someone or something triggers me. For example, I've had to make personal boundaries around not consuming entertainment that includes graphic depictions of sexual violence, as I just can't handle it emotionally. Sometimes that also looks like setting limits with friends or situations that don't make me feel safe. For instance, I prefer not to spend time in bars around lots of people getting drunk. I would rather risk someone thinking I'm a weirdo or not going with their flow than feel destabilized.

When it comes to trauma and the grief that accompanies it, our conditioning is to repress them, along with any outward displays of suffering. Yet pain, loss, and mourning over what or whom we've lost or has been taken from us (including parts of ourselves scarred by trauma) are all natural human emotions that must be felt and expressed. The more we try to bury the scars, the more they blister and turn our void darker; make our anger, anxiety, fear, and depression deeper.

Other people may be as uncomfortable with our grief as they are with their own shame or avoidance of trauma. To be vulnerable sometimes means being loud, messy, and tearful. We may not allow ourselves to lose control, and this in turn makes us rigidly monitor our own feelings and memories of trauma when they resurface. For me, when I refuse to acknowledge or go to the pain because it's not convenient to release, past trauma often registers as a low-grade depression. Reality is, sometimes trauma memory interrupts our routine or disturbs the equilibrium of what we present to the world. But in a safe space, either with trusted loved ones or with a professional—and sometimes even alone if you feel able to—allowing uncomfortable feelings or memories to move through us, uncensored and unjudged, can be strangely soothing, even inspiring personal breakthroughs.

Sometimes trauma can mark a major positive turning point in our lives if we are able to reframe its power. The Mexican artist Frida Kahlo had a severe bus accident in 1925 during which an iron handrail pierced through her pelvis, fracturing her pelvis bone, puncturing her uterus and abdomen, breaking her spine in three places, and dislocating her shoulder. It also broke her collarbone, several vertebrae, and her right leg in eleven places.

While spending months recovering in a full body cast, Kahlo began to paint, using her own bandaged torso as canvas. Throughout her life, she wore plaster corsets to help support her spine from this life-altering accident. You can still see some of the incredible artwork she created from her orthopedic corsets, which belong to the collection of La Casa Azul, the Frida Kahlo Museum in Mexico City.

I thought a lot about Frida Kahlo's cast paintings when I had a freak accident in my garden that landed me in the hospital with a compound fracture of my tibia, fibula, and ankle. The resulting emergency surgery, in which doctors inserted a permanent metal rod and four screws in my right leg, was accompanied by heavy painkillers given intravenously in the hospital, which made me foggy and caused panic attacks. I spent the next four and a half months learning to walk again. It humbled me to my core and completely changed my life. For the better, as it turned out. I slowed down to focus completely on something I had taken for granted (being able-bodied) and learned how powerful it is to *be vulnerable*. For someone who always had trouble asking for or receiving help, suddenly I needed it to do the most basic tasks, from taking a shower to getting down a flight of stairs. I was initially embarrassed, and I remembered how my father and the many older people I had been around toward the end of their lives reacted when their ability to fend for themselves was taken away. Then I thought about how we protect and nurture babies. We don't think twice about cleaning their diapers, wiping their assholes, or worrying about spit spewed on our clothes in a fit of colic as we hold them. We accept these human messes without judgment. We will gladly clean up a baby's shit with *love*.

Interestingly, the way men reacted to my damsel-in-distress vibe also showed me what a blessing vulnerability is. I couldn't tell you how many suitors I had while I was in recovery! They were literally knocking down my door, bringing me presents, cooking meals, and doing dishes for me. My DMs anytime I posted a picture with my fitted orthopedic stocking and Birkenstocks—items I previously would have been horrified to wear—were full of effusive messages from fetishists.

Our traumas are a part of us; they don't need to be our defining characteristic, but they are scars we carry. Healing and self-discovery (including around our sexuality) are lifelong processes, and the more we accept the point on the journey we are on right *now*, the less we beat ourselves up over where we *think we should be* or what we have suffered in the past.

Mykki Blanco is an internationally renowned performance artist, LGBTQIA+ and HIV+ activist, and musician who's worked with the likes of Bjork, Madonna, Kathleen Hanna, Kanye West, Major Lazer, and more, in addition to their solo career. Mykki told me, **"I just come from this background of hardcore trauma. One thing about becoming enlightened about something is that once [awareness] happens, it's never too late. And once healing happens, it changes everything. All the cells in your body and all the nucleuses and atoms in your body shift, and you're like, 'Wow, I've had a whole paradigm shift.'"**

The lessons we learn from traumas can end up being some of our greatest strengths, marks of the warrior who has metabolized the experiences from the battlefield. Facing our trauma, when and if we are ready to, can provide a massive reset in our conditioned responses to love, sex, and intimacy. It is not easy work to dig into the depths of our past pain, but the upside can be that we create a new story, a new way of relating to and loving ourselves and others—that is, if we can accept the parts of ourselves that we think are "broken" as essential to what makes us who we are. And if we can love these parts of ourselves, can we love the parts of our lovers that are scarred, too? Can we be gentle on ourselves and our partners and understand when they or we don't want to be sexual because we are consumed by loss? Can we hold space for sex that is nurturing and healing? Can we give support to other people in our lives and communities who may be healing from their traumas? Could we find alternatives to "How are you?" and "I'm fine"? Could we all admit that we aren't okay but are doing our best, at this moment right now, and we need a little support?

Here are some further resources to help on your journey.

National Suicide Prevention Lifeline
suicidepreventionlifeline.org/talk-to-someone-now/
800-273-8255

OpenCounseling International Suicide Hotlines
opencounseling.com/suicide-hotlines

Rape, Abuse & Incest National Network (RAINN)
rainn.org
1-800-656-HOPE (4673)

Substance Abuse and Mental Health Services Administration (SAMHSA)
samhsa.gov
800-662-HELP (4357)

BOUNDARIES, BONDAGE, AND HEALING

D o you know what your boundaries are around sex and love? What about your boundaries for touch, intimacy, relationships? Have you named your boundaries aloud? Have you communicated them to partners, friends, or family members? Are your boundaries being met?

When we lack healthy boundaries, our self-esteem suffers. We may find it hard to speak up when something doesn't feel right, whether in a sexual encounter or a friendship or a family dynamic. We may not know how to honor our feelings or what we need to receive in a relationship in order to feel seen and heard. Often we unconsciously place the needs of others above our own. This takes us out of a grounded place of empowerment when it comes to making decisions around sex.

Many of us were given literally zero guidance on how to recognize and set boundaries from the time we were kids. We grew up feeling like we had no right to have boundaries around our own bodies, told to "hug and kiss your grandma/cousin/uncle" whether or not we felt comfortable doing so. As adults, we are faced with someone coming in for a hug or a cheek kiss whether or not we invited it. It's almost like our physical boundaries are seen as permeable, as based on what someone else's social expectations are.

When we start experimenting sexually, we don't spend much time thinking about or learning how to communicate with a partner about what we are okay with and what we aren't. Even if we have received some kind of consent-based sex education, when we are faced with an intimate encounter as adolescents, the experience is more like trial by fire. This is also a time when we may be especially influenced by peer pressure and the urge to people please. That can last well into our twenties and beyond, particularly for women, who have been ingrained with cultural subliminal messages to *be polite* and a *caretaker.*

There is a common gesture many boys unconsciously use, generation after generation. They push someone's head down to nonverbally signal "I want a blow job." I was on the receiving end of this sign language more than once as a teenager. Sometimes it was easier to go along than to say, "I don't want to" or "Lick my pussy, then we'll talk." It took me a long time to develop the skills to name my boundaries aloud, and in many instances outside of the bedroom I still have to make sure I am sticking to them.

Understanding what our boundaries and needs are in a relationship and asserting that they be met can be incredibly difficult. People around us may be challenged when we compassionately relate our expectations and what doesn't fly. They may push back and react against them, especially if they aren't used to you asserting expectations. We can be so clear in *knowing* what we deserve—reciprocal nurturing, respect, an equilibrium of give and take—and yet find ourselves lacking the confidence to verbalize our requests or repeatedly feeling like we are coming up short.

Explicitly understanding our boundaries and how they apply to our relationships—notably sexual and romantic ones—takes a lot of discipline. If you've ever had to do physical therapy, you might know how frustrating and uncomfortable some of the exercises are. For example, you may be required to repeatedly move your big toe up and down. It seems so inconsequential but ends up affecting your entire mobilization and walking pattern. The good news is that if we can push past the fear and hesitation around honoring our boundaries, we can set new patterns that lead to richer, more fulfilling relationships all around.

In order to foster intimate relationships that come from a place of self-esteem and self-love, it is essential that we communicate our boundaries, even if it means having an awkward conversation or risking the possibility that someone cannot deliver on what we are asking for. Maintaining boundaries may cause some relationships to drop off if people are unable to meet you where you are, but it will also open up space for new ones to come in.

I spend the bulk of my time listening to and fielding questions from people about their most intimate lives. I need to be able to hold space for others' trauma and confusion around sexuality. Until I learned to create boundaries,

I would end my days drained and depressed over all the suffering I was taking in. I don't want to stop doing my work, so boundary setting is essential in order for me to be able to do what I love: helping bring light and information around the subject of sexuality so that we can heal this part of ourselves. Personally, the more I continue my own healing work around sex, love, and all kinds of relationship dynamics, the more I believe in *setting radical boundaries* and *practicing radical self-care*. These practices include having clear limits on my time and energy, cutting out people and places that don't make me feel good, and prioritizing activities that feed me on a deep level.

When it comes to sex, whether it is vanilla or extreme, it is especially important to be aware of your boundaries and self-care rituals. The safer you feel, the more you can let yourself go. Being sober of mind when engaging in high-risk sexual activities for the first time and/or with a new partner (bondage, choking,[12] group sex, and more) is critical. Our boundaries slip when we are high or drunk, becoming blurred all too easily.

In kink- and fetish-friendly communities and relationships, it is common practice for boundaries to be negotiated explicitly before any consensual sexual activity takes place. Nina Hartley elaborates:

> We don't just end up holding a whip or being whipped. You negotiate. What does this mean to us? What is this building between us? In our culture, sex just happens. It's like you don't end up naked. Choices were made. They could be unconscious choices. They could be unhealthful choices. They can be unaware choices. But choices were made before you [found] yourself naked in someone's bed.
>
> For everyone's health and also to reduce instances of harassment or assault, as adults, [the period] between impulse and action, we spread that out as long as necessary so everyone's safe and happy. So, the impulse: "Ooh, I would love to get to know you better." Instead of, "Tomorrow night," say, "Hey, let's sit down and have coffee with our clothes on. You may need to be in a relationship, and I may want to have a playmate, so we'll have to just stick to coffee."

---

12   Consensual choking should not be practiced high or drunk by either party. It is imperative you are facing your partner, as breathing and lack of oxygen need to be monitored. You cannot see someone turning blue if they are facing away from you. I am flooded with questions about choking from people born post-1990 (and their parents) who received the bulk of their sex modeling from streaming pornography.

For grown-up people who want to have better sex more often, extend the time between mutual expression of desire and actual action as long as necessary to have any conversation needed so that you and I both feel really great about it. The negotiation is setting the shape of the playground. The spontaneity will fill in the playground. "You got a job, and I got a kid." We can set aside a time in which spontaneity can certainly be promoted. But the idea that it was going to be spontaneous, that's unrealistic.

The late Mistress Velvet, who passed away in 2021, was Chicago's premier African dominatrix. Velvet had been practicing risk-aware consensual kink since 2014, and their domination was rooted in black femme supremacy. They were known for making their white male submissives read black feminist theory and pay symbolic reparations. Velvet told me that they had to create

a lot of boundaries at the end of the session. I do a lot of work before a session to get myself into the role of Mistress Velvet, which ties into my literal preparation, my makeup and doing my hair, but I'll also listen to certain music. [Afterward] I have to do things like that to leave her in the dungeon. I never really want [my clients] to see me outside of being Mistress Velvet, but sometimes that happens. Let's say they went to take a shower and I'm wiping up the dungeon. When I start cleaning the bed, for example, I really leave that headspace, because I'm like, "Okay, now I have these things I need to do." And so I've had clients come talk to me, and they were just chitchatting like normal people, which I think they really, really love, but it makes it very confusing for me. I usually create some routines. I'll go have dinner by myself, which makes me feel very vulnerable. Usually during that time I will reflect on the session.

I think of sex work as a form of caretaking. I'm definitely [taking on the role of my client's] therapist, so I have to also take care of myself if I want to be there for them in the way that I want.

If you've read this far, I know you have an open mind. So let's keep it that way for what I'm going to tell you next: *rope play, bondage, and other forms of kink* may be extremely useful when it comes to learning what your boundaries are and how to communicate them clearly. Some people have also found bondage to be a helpful tool in trauma-healing work. Make sure to consult with a trusted professional if you have a history of trauma before exploring any of these modalities in a safe environment. As with anything when it comes to sexual activity, it is imperative that *you feel safe*.

I believe that we can learn a whole lot about how to behave in so-called heteronormative vanilla relationships from approaches practiced by the BDSM,[13] fetish, and kink communities. Beyond the exercise of communication and negotiating boundaries, two concepts that I believe should be applied to all sexual encounters, even the most casual hookups, are *aftercare* and *subspace*.

Subspace is an altered state of consciousness brought on by the hormones—adrenaline and endorphins—rushing through your body and brain post–sexual play. Subspace is different for every person and every situation. We can all agree that whether it is intense, amazing, painful, or so-so, engaging in a sexual act with another human being does have some kind of impact on our psyche, right? You feel very different before and after an orgasm. On a physical level you might be completely exhausted and need to pass out or exhilarated with endless energy and ready to go again. Emotionally you could be experiencing a multitude of feelings ranging from joy to grief. Regardless of the specifics, you are in a temporary state—kind of like being drunk or high—and it will take a moment to recalibrate back to your baseline "normal."

Aftercare is how you and your partner show care and kindness postrendezvous. You've just participated in an intimate act and/or intense sexual experience. Now that it is over, you are not going to forget to be compassionate and communicative, right? Aftercare helps each party to feel that the consensual sex act they were just involved in was special. We are not talking about defining relationship status; we are simply being mindful of what was just shared. This applies to a one-night stand or a longstanding relationship.

In the BDSM, fetish, and kink communities, an intimate encounter (whether or not it includes penetrative sex) is usually referred to as a "scene." The action of the dominant party is "topping," and the submissive's, "bottoming." As Dr. Wendy Cherry says, **"After a scene with a dominant/submissive**

---

13   Encompassing a vast array of acts and communities, this abbreviation roughly stands for "bondage/discipline, dominance/submission, and sadism/masochism." In this sexual terrain, the consensual adoption of amplified power-dynamic play is the turn-on, and a "safe word" keeps all aware of the limits. Controlled pain, restriction, sensory deprivation, subordinance, and worship are among the range of kinks discussed by partners ahead of time in order to establish boundaries.

pairing, the submissive is nurtured, held, wiped down, cradled, cuddled, and given water. They are taken care of because they've just really gone on a transcendent spiritual journey."

I hear from so many people in heteronormative vanilla or casual relationships who would really appreciate an aftercare experience. It is okay to tell someone that you'd like to hear from them postsex, just a check-in within twenty-four hours, *if that is what you need.* This is setting a healthy boundary for yourself and honoring your body. It is a very basic form of human politeness and consideration—especially if someone just sucked your cock, licked your ass, or ate your pussy!

I had a conversation about why aftercare is so important with Midori, a legendary sex educator, author, and artist. Midori wrote the first English-language book on *shibari, The Seductive Art of Japanese Bondage,* which has become the classic rope bible. She stressed how important it is that one

discuss one's need for aftercare in advance. If you and I were playing and you were somebody who wanted an intense degree of physical touch to come back to your equilibrium, and I'm somebody who needed alone-ness to regain my equilibrium—if we didn't talk about this in advance and we have an amazing playtime and that comes to an end and then I get up and walk away, you would feel abandoned. And I would feel smothered if you were draped over me and touching me a lot if I were an "I need to be alone" person. If we discovered this in advance, here's what I might do. I'm going to spend some time with you, for your aftercare, but in my head I'm going to consider it part of my scene. At a certain point, I'm going to have to leave, and it's because we had a good time and I actually need to reintegrate.

Now most of the time, people don't ask about what they need for aftercare. If they did, it would save them a lot of grief. This applies to all sexual experiences. A lot of it has to do with brain chemicals—the high and pleasure from good sex can last forty-eight hours. And then when you come out of that you can have a crash and feel all sad.

Even though I am someone who counts among her close friends and colleagues many people who engage in bondage, fetish, and rope play, for many years I had little to no practical experience. Over the course of our thirteen-year relationship, my ex-husband and I had experimented as amateurs with binding hands, blindfolds, and spanking, but I'd never been professionally bound. I was a true "rope virgin." I kept hearing about how bondage could be incredibly empowering and healing. Many of my friends who worked in this space said that the bulk of their clients were people, mainly women, working through high degrees of sexual trauma to reclaim their bodies and sense of trust. It wasn't until I was tied up by a master of the craft that my body and mind truly appreciated the awesome transformative power that bondage could bring.

I have been friends for many years with Betony Vernon, who is a sexual anthropologist, erotic jeweler, author, and "mastress" of the ropes. We met in the early 2000s through the fashion world in Paris, where she designed a gorgeous basement-level salon, a wraparound iron staircase leading down to a hidden world of pleasure and luxury. I'm talking cherrywood, green velvets, leather sex furniture, and display cabinets full of her shiny erotic jewelry. Next-level Parisian chic.

Betony was based in Europe, and I was living in Los Angeles. We spoke often about our respective work, and many times over the course of a decade, she suggested that I should experience being bound and offered to show me the ropes, so to speak. Finally, we scheduled a session, and it turned out that our timing was just right. My father had just died, and I was grieving his loss, feeling particularly vulnerable.

At the time, my boundaries were extremely malleable, and I struggled to honor and vocalize what did and did not feel "right" to me when it came to relationships, intimate and otherwise. I hear so many people say they "should know this" or "should have learned by now" when it comes to boundaries or sex, but let this story be a lesson in how someone can have all the access to information and intellectual understanding I thought I did and still fail themselves in the moment when it comes to speaking up. *This is okay and totally normal.* Hindsight is 20/20, right? Add to the mix the heavy grief and destabilization I was undergoing, and it's no wonder I wasn't feeling grounded or empowered.

The plan was to meet in Betony's hotel room in Los Angeles, share tea, and have her tie me up. We would be joined by a mutual close friend who also had a couple of decades' experience in the bondage and fetish space, as well as another woman I didn't know well and had never felt comfortable with. But I didn't speak up. I felt intimidated by their collective years of, let's call it, non-vanilla-sex professional and personal experience, and I didn't want to come across as an insecure newbie. To coordinate the agenda, we had a group text going. I made a joke of my inexperience, texting the others, "I feel like a sacrificial lamb with the hot Witches of Eastwick" instead of privately telling Betony or my close friend how tender I felt.

This was the first boundary of mine I discredited in this situation. My body knew something was off, but my mind pushed my doubts aside in favor of "What would they think?" or "How might they judge me?" Unfortunately this happens a lot when it comes to our instincts. Those little "off" feelings are really important to listen to. I'm not an exhibitionist, and I am honestly quite shy naturally. Not when it comes to public speaking or working a room, but in intimate situations, I am one raw, sensitive nerve. So having an audience watching me while experiencing something I was already anxious about added an extra layer of pressure.

Betony started to bind me in an intricate, magnificent corset made entirely of rope, wrapping it around my breasts, rib cage, and spine like a constricting spiderweb. As she wound the hemp cords round and round, tighter with each knot, I found it hard to breathe. Each time my shoulders rose and I froze up, she would stop, look me in the eyes, and repeat, "Feel your body, remember your yoga practice, remember to breathe." Together, we would take several long breaths until I felt calm and ready to continue.

Have you ever been too much in your head to let go sexually? Being tightly bound, my breath restricted by the ropes, forced me to focus and ground into my body and the experience. I had to stay present to feel where my edges were. And keep breathing to prevent passing out.

The act of creating the corset went on for over an hour, after which she led me around the room by the ends of the ropes knotted at the back of my spine. She told me to look at myself in the hotel room mirror, to admire how beautiful I looked, the rope corset accentuating my curves. At the time, I was embarrassed by the idea of admiring myself. Yet while writing this chapter, I discovered Polaroid photographs from this session, and I have to say, I looked amazing! I found it hard to relax, feeling extremely self-conscious, especially with three people watching me, but Betony made me feel safe as she prompted me again and again to *stay present*. I trusted her enough to allow myself to be led by her capable hands. She was in total command.

Together, we tested the limits of how much constriction I could handle. I was okay with the rope corset and my hands being tied, but the moment she suggested binding both my legs or a hogtie—legs and arms bound together behind the back, lying prone on the floor, like a pig ready for slaughter—I immediately seized up. My body screamed, "NO!" and I honored that. I was grateful a professional was helping me navigate my bondage boundaries and respecting them, instead of working this out, amateur style, with some fuckboy.

After we established my comfort level, or baseline, for rope play, she pulled out some of the erotic accessories she designed, among them a silver-handled horsehair whip and an ostrich feather tickler. Seriously, the ultimate luxury erotic accessories one could hope to have in their bedroom. It was fun having Betony show me how they worked, but with the extra audience sitting on the couch watching me, I couldn't fully let go.

At one point Betony asked my permission to leave the room to use the bathroom. I gave my consent. As soon as she left, the other two women started making jokes about using some of the other erotic objects on me. There was a silver butt plug that I had expressed to Betony in front of all parties I was not interested in trying in this setting. My close friend picked it up and came up to me, laughing about how she was going to use it. The other woman was laughing, too; they were egging each other on. I was the sacrificial lamb—yet I had put myself in that position, no one to blame but myself.

I was feeling defenseless, my body and hands tightly bound. I couldn't move freely, as Betony had placed me kneeling on a settee. Betony, my "caretaker," had left the room for a few moments, and now I had an overwhelming feeling of helplessness—and I was completely unable to verbalize it to my friend. For her, it was no big deal to play in this space, so why should it be for me? Instead of recognizing my boundaries or saying aloud, "I am really uncomfortable, please stop," I tried to laugh along with them.

Thankfully, Betony came back into the room and took charge. She could see that I was ready to be liberated from the ropes, as it had been several hours by now. She asked if, before she released me, I would like to try a trust exercise.

Did you ever play that trust-fall game when you were a kid? The one where you have to fall backward into someone's arms and let them catch you? There I was, bound in this gorgeous rope corset, enveloped from collarbone to crotch, with all the knots meeting at the center of my back. Betony held the connecting ends of the ropes in her hands. She asked me, instead of falling backward, to fall forward. Before I hit the floor, she pulled the cords taut so I was suspended, hovering above the ground. There was a massive shift in my body. I felt safe, supported, like I could completely *trust in my body to let go and be held.*

The ropes guarded my limbs in a womb-like embrace. I was reduced to an infant state of consciousness, bound by a rope umbilical cord. Betony, as my caretaker and domme,[14] was a nurturing force, responsible for my safety and well-being with my cords in her hands. It was the first time I knew *in my body* how beneficial bondage could be for reclaiming trust and confidence in my boundaries. I realize this experience may not work for everyone, but it had an overwhelmingly positive effect on me, perhaps because I experienced it with someone I was able to be vulnerable with, safely.

A conscious dom/sub[15] power exchange allows responsibility and vulnerability, much like the relationship between a primary caregiver and an infant. Ideally, a caregiver's priority is to feed, bathe, love, play with, nourish, and protect a child at all costs. Historically, this is not the experience for a large population on the planet. So many children and adults from families around the world grow up without having this basic human need to be nurtured fulfilled.

We unconsciously learn boundaries and how we attach in relationships from our earliest caretakers. The psychological term *attachment style* refers to a theory of how we relate to other humans. Attachment styles generally fall into one of four categories: secure, anxious-preoccupied, dismissive-avoidant, and fearful-avoidant. During our first year of life, our particular style is determined by how our needs are met (or ignored) by our primary caregiver(s). Our attachment style contributes to our defense mechanisms (for example, building walls around ourselves, needing constant reassurance), the way we love, and how we behave in romantic relationships.

Many mental health professionals and sexual therapists speculate that we unconsciously choose romantic partners in order to recreate a relationship that is similar to one we had with the parent or parents of conflict, for the purposes of repairing our childhood. We tend to do it over and over. However, we

---

14 *Domme* is the feminine short form of *dominant* (*dom* being the masculine form). All these terms describe those who hold and exert the majority of power within any relationship (sexual, romantic, or otherwise). It is important to note that all parameters of the relationship have been discussed and negotiated prior to "playing" (starting a relationship) between partners.

15 This term refers to a person who, within the BDSM community, relinquishes control in a power-exchange dynamic. Submissives are encouraged to discuss their boundaries in the form of "hard" (absolutely not) and "soft" (maybe, if I feel more comfortable) no's during negotiation (as are dominants). Conventionally, the role has been equated with the "bottom," but a submissive can take on many roles (and positions!) in accordance with their dominant's/dominants' directions (and previously discussed negotiations).

don't have to repeat the patterns if we recognize and accept these hurt parts of ourselves. If we want to change our paradigm, bondage can be useful for reconnecting to the caregiver experience in a loving, protected space we may have never known as infants. Again, please check with a professional therapist if you are using bondage work as a healing modality post–sexual assault, as you will need extra care and the right support to work through the feelings that arise.

Later, Betony told me that she does a lot of breakthrough and healing work:

> I enter contracts much like what we did together, which wasn't erotic. I mean, it is erotic because it is the body. But the only thing I asked you to do was to come feeling beautiful, and you did. It is about connecting the mind to the body, and *trust is really fundamental, because if you don't trust someone, then you can't really let go* [emphasis mine]. The cords, if you lean into them and you give way to them, are all about letting go. Once you're set free, you realize that there has been a shift. The brain goes into a mode that is a little bit on alert, just because it's not normal to be constricted, and it's not normal to be hugged, especially the first time. I consider when I'm doing healing sessions that the cords are like a hug that takes over your whole body. I have a method where I tie you into a tight, sort-of fetal position that's elaborate, and at the end, I set you free with scissors. It creates a release response, which is powerful.
>
> *It's about building trust again, trust in others, trust in your own body, and trust in the cords, and feeling connected* [emphasis mine]. From a symbolic point of view, we are connected to the cord, which is the umbilical cord as [if] we are children, and so I try to bring that symbolism into my technique in healing sessions.

Around the same time as my session with Betony, a male friend shared with me that when he was a child playing a trust game with his father, his father let him fall, saying, "Let that be a lesson. Never trust anyone." He was traumatized and subsequently had difficulty finding fulfilling intimate relationships. He wasn't shown as a child that he could count on the people closest to him for support—in fact, he learned the opposite. I remember thinking how amazing it was that experiencing safety and trust during rope play could allow one to reclaim the parts of themselves that had been scarred.

After Betony unbound me, I felt an imprint, "ghost ropes," on my skin for days afterward. Instead of going to dinner with the group, I went home and cried. I was dating someone new at this time, and when I told him about the experience, instead of asking me how I had felt, he was both titillated and freaked out by me doing something he considered "dirty." He didn't see it as I did, as an exercise in healing, trust, and self-empowerment.

It took a while to process my first bondage experience, and even writing about it years later, I am enlightened by aspects I didn't recognize at the time. I never would have thought that it would be such a huge lesson for me in respecting and verbalizing my boundaries. Or that it would illuminate how often I ignored "off" feelings or wasn't present in my body during sexual situations. I can now take accountability for naming what does and doesn't feel good, both in intimate relationships and outside of them.

I am so grateful to Betony for busting my bondage cherry and continuing to teach me the myriad ways that cords can be used in times of deep healing. Long after this first encounter, she and I worked together again, after the breakup of a committed relationship with someone I deeply loved. This time we did a session with just the two of us, in my home. Instead of using hemp ropes, she had me pick out fifty yards of silk ribbon in a color that I felt represented me. As she wrapped me up in another intricate, yet this time soft, braided pink corset, she repeatedly said, "Look at you. You are so beautiful. You are a gift." She reminded me to fetishize *myself.* To center from a place of empowerment, with deep love and honor for my body. To view my sexuality as a sacred temple and treasure, to be held in the highest esteem. To choose partners from a position of self-love and with clear boundaries.

Bondage, done with a professional or someone you trust and are able to communicate honestly with, can heighten the intersection of spirituality and sexuality and lead to transcendent erotic experiences. Being restrained increases mind-body awareness, allowing us to be fully present and grounded in a sensual experience. Being bound can also help us clarify boundaries, both physically and emotionally.

My boundaries may look completely different from yours, just like our sexuality does. While I may need a gentle, less-is-more touch to feel at ease, you might prefer to be suspended by ropes, hogtied, and flogged to let go. Neither is a right or wrong approach. It is about finding what works for you, letting go of judgments regarding what other people's needs and limits may be, and respecting them, too.

Here are some exercises to help honor your boundaries.

1. Only you know what feels appropriate, and only you have the power to claim your personal space. One way to get comfortable with this is to take a few minutes at the start of the day with a simple visualization. Close your eyes and imagine a protective bubble of light around you; it can be any color, shape, or size you desire. Then stand in this space you've created. Acknowledge it. OWN IT.

   Sometimes when I need extra protection—for example, if I am going to be in an intense environment or dealing with people I don't particularly trust (hey, life happens)—I will spend extra time interior designing my bubble, with chic 1960s space-age Barbie decor and a sheepskin rug. I get real comfortable there until I feel like it's my safe place. I wrap that light all around me! You can even open your eyes and create a physical field around you using your hands or any movements. Get creative!

2. Name your needs. Make a list. This can include your needs in a romantic, sexual, or platonic relationship. Naming these needs to yourself will then help you name them aloud to others. When you're ready, it could be as simple as saying to a friend, "I really need a hug" or "I need to know that what I tell you stays between us." You could state what you need to feel comfortable having sex with a new partner: "I need us to share STI test results before we discuss not using condoms." Or you might say to a regular lover, "I don't like having X touched" or "I want to talk to you on the phone three times a week."

3. It is okay to communicate when your boundaries are being challenged. For example, you could say, "I felt really uncomfortable when you insisted I should try X because you like it" or "Please stop pressuring me into telling you intimate details about my sex life."

   Sometimes we are not able to communicate with the person who violated our boundaries, either because it is unsafe or because time and circumstances do not permit. In this case, write down how you felt your boundaries were violated and, if you feel comfortable, share it with someone you trust or a therapist.

4. Practice becoming comfortable with clear phrases like "No," "Please don't," "I feel disrespected when . . . ," or "I'm not available."

5. If you want people to respect your boundaries, you must respect theirs. You could ask, "I'm so turned on by you and want to give you pleasure. How do you like to be touched? Are there areas that I should avoid?" This may feel awkward at first, but I promise you, the more you do it the more confident you will feel and the easier it will get.

6. Acknowledge when you disrespect someone else's boundaries. For example, someone has asked you explicitly not to divulge private conversations they have with you. You do it anyway, and it gets back to them. Instead of denying or acting like it's no big deal, take responsibility for your lack of consideration to the boundary they established with you.

Boundaries will positively change your relationships and sex life. It is not too late to start verbalizing and setting them—or changing existing ones—right now. Some people may not be able to accept a new relationship dynamic, but others may surprise you with their willingness to evolve as you do. We may need to relearn our boundaries over and over as we interact with different people and situations; this is totally normal and to be expected. What we want to aim for is creating safe containers for our relationships, be they romantic, familial, business, or platonic, so we can appropriately express the truest version of ourselves within these contexts.

Do you want to incorporate some of the ethics from fetish and kink into casual or monogamous relationships? Can we all agree that transactional sex could benefit from the basic etiquette of aftercare? Are we ready to evolve how we *communicate* around sex?

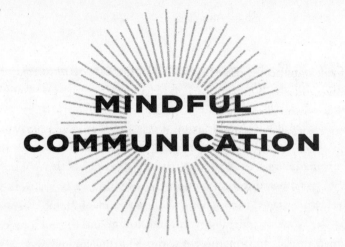

MINDFUL COMMUNICATION

You'd think for a writer with two books under her garters, a chapter on mindful communication would just flow forth. Instead, I'm hit by realizations about when I've failed to communicate clearly, how I could have communicated more effectively, and the many times I didn't actively listen.

Contemplating my relationships—romantic, familial, friendly—I see countless details (and red flags) I overlooked even though people told them to me up front. Important things I left out or avoided verbalizing.

I recall innumerable lies I told myself or others because I was afraid to be authentic and vulnerable. Afraid of being judged, of not being accepted, of sharing something intimate and receiving a response I didn't like.

I know I'm not the only one who bottles things up rather than admit an embarrassing truth.

While writing this chapter, I had a conversation with an ex that enlightened me about how unsuccessful we were at communicating as a couple. I had gone silent on him after discovering a repeated lie we had gone over multiple times in the relationship, needing some space to gain clarity. He told me he had tried to "communicate" with me repeatedly—which in this case meant I received three emoji texts (a sad face, tears, and a shrug) and a couple of missed calls with no voice message. Is this communicating? What happens when one or both parties engage in passive-aggressive communication like we did? Could I have done a better job of expressing myself to him? When we avoid naming the thing that upsets us about a situation or relationship, no one has the chance to evolve. Is it possible that we don't know how to listen to *ourselves* in order to speak our truths aloud?

Cut to postbreakup: we had an honest conversation in which he revealed to me that he often lies to "avoid saying something that would hurt someone I love." Does this work? Have you done this yourself? Have I? It made me think about how many of us avoid relating truthfully to one another out of fear.

We don't get much direction on how to communicate honestly. In fact, we are actively discouraged from talking about most uncomfortable, complicated subjects—sex, death, vulnerability, mental health, and so much more. These very human topics can bring up conscious and unconscious shame, whether our own or what others may project onto us. Our collective lack of practice in being in touch with our feelings and knowing how to mindfully communicate them holds us back from being honest with ourselves and the people we love.

Of all the subjects in the world, one that seems especially challenging for people to communicate freely about is sex.[16] Despite all our access to sex in the digital age, we have very little modeling around how to have IRL (not digital) relationships, to have great sex, or to be truly intimate. Much of this is due to awkwardness in finding the right language to express our deepest desires and vulnerabilities.

We spend a lot of time supposedly "communicating," sending thousands of emails, delivering DMs and PMs across platforms, posting comments on social media. It's second nature to "like" a text, send a meme, or type "K" (even if it's not).

If you use hookup or dating apps, you encounter even more nuanced language to sort through: "u up? WYD? DTF?" It's exhausting just thinking about how much we "communicate" on a daily basis. But are we actually communicating?

Our dependency on devices and their shorthand means we lack practice in the art and subtlety of conscious communication. Compare the amount and quality of your intimate face-to-face conversations with the number of people you have "communicated" with via devices today. What about this week, month, year? Do you notice a discrepancy?

It turns out that 90 percent of human communication is nonverbal. So many subtleties get lost in digital communication: our scents, body language,

---

16 And death, but we will get into that later.

whether we look each other in the eyes or avoid eye contact—all this extra information we could be absorbing behind the words being spoken. Details that inform how we express ourselves and how we take in what other people are saying.

Even when we are communicating face-to-face, there's often a huge difference between what we verbalize and what we really think and feel. I can speak in public with relative nonchalance, but one-on-one conversations—small talk especially—is challenging for me. Often I feel like I have a mask on, usually aided by red lipstick, to assume a different version of myself. One that can produce more confident, effortless chatter. Performative communication, if you will.

How does one even go about creating mindful communication? It starts with noticing how you are feeling. Let's take, for example, a scenario with a family member with whom you have a strained relationship. Are you feeling offensive or defensive before either of you open your mouths? Are you planning your rebuttal in your head while they are speaking, or are you actively listening? Or let's say you're in a monogamous relationship and your partner tells you that they are having feelings for someone else. Do you feel hurt, rejected, angry? Do you dismiss the conversation or shut it down completely because the reality is just too upsetting to face? Or are you the one who is attracted to someone else but is afraid to verbalize it to your partner? Does not acknowledging it mean those desires are gone?

Just noticing, alone, how *you* feel can impact the words you choose to express. The goal is to notice when you are using resentment, punishment, or avoidance as a defense against being vulnerable. If we can stay centered in vulnerability, we may be able to achieve greater clarity when expressing ourselves. Our ability to recognize what is going on inside of us and communicate it improves all our relationships, whether romantic or platonic.

Have you ever told a lie about how sexually fulfilled you were by a partner? Are you telling yourself that lie right now? Did you or have you expressed aloud that you were not fulfilled to the other person? Are you unsure how?

Recently, a heterosexual man in his thirties, just out of a long-term relationship, told me that he and his partner had always come together. Every. Single. Time. Oh, honey. I wonder if his ex thought she was doing him a favor by faking an orgasm. I mean, I've done it, too—but ultimately we don't get the rewards (better sex for all parties) if we don't confront the challenge of an awkward conversation. The truth may sting a bit, but if it comes from a loving place, it is always better to state it, and it always leads to more intimacy.

Someone sticking their tongue, fingers, penis, or strap-on[17] inside your orifices is a very intimate act . . . yet sometimes it can be even *more intimate* to talk about it.

Are you bored with the sex you are having but don't know what to do about it? Have you asked your partner about their fantasies? Have they asked about yours? Have you ever visited a sex shop together? Salespeople are trained to answer questions and make suggestions; it can be fun to browse, too. Kind of like going to an exotic car showroom. Sometimes you just need to give each other permission to expand your sexual repertoire. We can't expect the same old same old is going to work forever. It is important to continuously have these conversations and be open to what your partner is thinking about—without judgment.[18]

Are you sleeping with someone new? When were you and your partner(s) last tested? Are you exclusively sleeping with each other? What kind of protection are you using? Do you have an allergy to latex condoms? Are there places you like to be touched and others that are no-go zones? No one is a mind reader. The more we understand our own and our partners' desires, the more room we have to play and explore. Naming our boundaries aloud helps us let go of sexual inhibitions that may be holding us back from the most mind-blowing orgasms we could conceive.

Communication, honesty, and checking in with each other regularly about what is and isn't working are essential in sexual relationships of any kind. This includes asking each other questions and bringing up sticky subjects that we are trained to sweep under the rug.

Many people share with me their belief that sex is supposed to just "happen" magically and perfectly. As though talking about it aloud before you do it takes the excitement and mystery away; as though, if the person or timing is right, sex will just "work." Where did we get this fairy-tale idea that love, relationships, and sex are meant to be flawless if we and our partners are the "right fit"? Does having to struggle, overcome obstacles, and maneuver through inexperience make love

---

17 This is a term for a pelvically harnessed dildo, utilized by those without a penis (or without a penis capable of sustaining a satisfactory erection) for the purpose of sexually penetrating another. Most often associated with mainstream lesbian sex, cis straight couples have adopted its use more regularly with the growing acceptance of "pegging" (a woman anally penetrating a man).

18 As always, as long as it is with consent and doesn't involve minors or people who aren't able to give consent.

and sex any less amazing? Why is articulating our fears, desires, and insecurities so embarrassing when it comes to romantic or sexual situations?

Does anything in life just "work"? Like a mental movie, I imagine an outcome (such as finishing this book) and then I want to fast-forward to a completed draft that is immediately celebrated by my publisher. But instead, I have to slog through the writing process, step-by-step, not knowing how it's going to turn out. Just as any creative endeavor requires a certain amount of trust, energy, and risk, so too do love and intimacy. It takes constant communication and effort to achieve the rewards of great sex and enduring love.

Communicating about sex *before* we have it can expand our pleasure potential and enjoyment. The clearer we are and the better we express ourselves, the more successfully we can design an optimal playground for pleasure. Verbalizing in advance what we are turned on by as well as our boundaries also clears up miscommunication and unspoken assumptions that could potentially lead to sticky situations.

When I was a teenager and first experimenting sexually, there was absolutely no discussion, collectively or privately, about consent.[19] Now it's a buzzword filling our screens and lexicons, but how do we go about negotiating and implementing consent in real life? This is another reason why having what may feel like uncomfortable conversations *before* being naked (and potentially high or drunk) is essential. I hear a lot of "But what am I supposed to do? Ask every five minutes if I can do X, Y, or Z?" In the heat of the moment, rational thought often goes out the window. Here's where enthusiastic consent comes in, meaning that you establish an affirmative yes or "I like that, it feels good" instead of looking for a no, which can be hard for some people (especially those who are younger or suffering from low self-esteem) to voice.

The actor and comedian Nick Kroll told me that the concept of enthusiastic consent has played a big role in the writers' room of the Netflix animated show

---

19 Consent is the permission, the green light, or the "Fuck, yes" for something to happen or the agreement to something that has been thoroughly communicated and discussed beforehand. If you're having trouble remembering all of the specifics, Planned Parenthood has a helpful acronym: FRIES stands for "freely given" (not coerced, manipulated, or tricked), "reversible" (a person can freely change their mind), "informed" (what is going to happen has been communicated and discussed), "enthusiastic" (we may not always have the energy to be little sex bunnies, but the desire, the freely given yes, should be there), and "specific." It should be noted that saying yes to a specific invitation does not imply you've said yes to doing anything else.

he cocreated, *Big Mouth*. Interestingly, it's also important in the advice he gives to teenage boy fans. As he relates,

> I say, enthusiastic consent is on all levels useful. One, it's sexy, from
> a purely selfish point of view, getting your partner to say they want
> to do something with you, and hearing that your partner wants to
> do the things that you want to do with them, is very sexy and also
> incredibly relieving of tension. And also on the other side of that,
> post–[Brett] Kavanaugh hearings, everyone's like, "What are our
> boys supposed to do?" Boys are supposed to find out what's okay to
> do. And then enjoy doing that or [accepting] that they can't do that.
> And then there's no gray area [regarding] what people said, what they
> thought they interpreted as [to] what was okay or not okay. We're
> supposed to talk about everything.

Have you ever heard the expression "When you assume, you make an 'ass' out of 'u' and 'me'"? Many of us, especially when it comes to romance and sex, tend to assume what other people are thinking, feeling, and experiencing. A lot of this is projection on our part—us projecting our belief system onto others. I call this "psychic sex." **"Psychic sex means you think the other person should be able to read your mind about what you want to feel and what is going to be pleasurable for you,"** says Lou Paget, the bestselling author of five books on sexuality and a certified sex educator who travels the world sharing accurate, practical information with honesty and accessibility.

We may have a sense of whether something feels good or bad to us. But how do we know what feels right or wrong or good or shitty to me or her or them? Have we spent any time asking, sharing, and actively listening? Lou points out that

> many times people will go along with something not really enjoying
> it. And then someone downloads faulty software. A skill set is
> knowing what you like and knowing what the other person likes.
> And many times people will touch the way they like to be touched.
> [Which may not be how your partner likes it.] I had one woman
> who said, "I just want him to be there. That's what I want." And her
> partner said, "I didn't know where 'there' was." And it was something

that if she had used her hands to guide his hands, it would be a completely different feedback loop.

The other thing, if you want to be able to guide someone, use one word. Don't use a whole sentence. "Lighter." "Softer." "Yes." A sentence such as "That's not really what I like" is going to be heard as criticism. That really shuts people down. What we know as sex educators is to give people an opening so that they feel heard, they feel understood, and they know that they have a voice in this entire equation.

The truth is, *it's superhot to talk to your lover about how you like to fuck them and what you want to do with them.*

How do we break the ice when it comes to having what we may feel will be delicate conversations? First off, I suggest having a clothing-on talk outside of the bedroom (or whatever location you are usually intimate in)—maybe over coffee or dinner or in a casual setting. Discussing your needs and wants in the middle of hot and heavy action creates a lot of pressure. Communicating face-to-face, with good eye contact, is essential. If possible, try to look at the person in their left eye, which corresponds to the emotional seat of our brain.

Another tip is to use words that center a positive experience instead of focusing on what you *don't* like. Starting a sentence with "I feel" can be an encouraging way to lead in—for example, "I feel especially turned on when you . . ." This fosters a more relaxed, open conversation than leading with "I really hate it when you . . ." When you're talking about sexuality or sexual contact especially, don't talk about what the person is or isn't doing or what they're doing wrong," recommends Dr. Wendy Cherry. "Talk about yourself." Wendy recalls a young couple she was counseling.

She said, "He's so perfect, except I can't stand the way he kisses me. What do I do?" I said, "Why don't you sit cross-legged on the bed in front of him and say, 'I'm going to kiss you like I like to be kissed'?" . . . It's like, "You know what, sweetheart? I've always fantasized about so-and-so. Do you know what makes me feel really good?" Sexuality is particular. So you have to have a really open dialogue, but talk about yourself. That encourages your partner to talk about themselves and what they prefer and what they like.

The concept of psychic sex can apply to all sorts of love and other relationship scenarios—and contribute to us making snap judgments about other people and their motivations. I hear all the time from people in new relationships (especially heternormative ones) who can't face having an open conversation about whether they both do or don't want kids or whether they are exclusive or monogamous because they fear "putting pressure" on their partner. It's easier to just assume they are on the same page, but that assumption can lead to problems.

For many of the questions we receive at The Sex Ed, the short answer is essentially a version of: "Communicate." Here are some recent examples: "How do I ask my partner for more sex?" "How do I talk to my partner about opening up our relationship?" "I don't like it when my partner does X. What do I do?" and "How do I say no to anal sex?"

Let's break down how we might approach one of these conversations. I'm going to tackle the anal sex query, as we get so many questions about this from hetero women who either are having it for their first time; don't want to, but their partner does; or are enduring the act, but it doesn't feel good.

If this is something you are categorically not interested in but your partner keeps asking for it, you can suggest trying it on them first. (An "I'll try it if you do.") You can begin with a butt plug (starting small and gradually going to bigger sizes), or you can try pegging,[20] using a strap-on dildo to penetrate them. The male prostate is a source of extreme pleasure—it is considered the equivalent of the G-spot in women. If your partner is completely turned off by the idea of a reciprocal experience, this very conversation will be sure to open their mind—and they may think twice about pressuring you if they aren't open to it themselves.

I got this idea from my dear friend Ana de la Reguera, an actress, producer, and activist. Among her many film and television roles, she created, writes, produces, and stars in a semiautobiographical TV show, *Ana*, on Comedy Central. She told me:

> In my midtwenties, I tried anal. I wanted it, but I couldn't, it was
> so painful. It was horrible. So I knew that was a thing that I didn't

---

20 This is the act of anal or vaginal penetration via the use of a strap-on (pelvically harnessed dildo). For those without penile anatomy, it allows for what many deem to be the adoption of the penetrative role between partners.

want to do. And then in my midthirties, I had this relationship, and he said, "I want to have anal sex" [all the time]. And at some point, I got tired [of him asking], so I said, "Okay. Let's have anal sex, but you go first. I'm going to put on a dildo and a belt, and you go first, and if you like it, I'll do it. We have to be even." And he didn't want to do it, and I was like, "Okay, so you don't want to do it. Then I don't want to do it either."

Bottom line (no pun intended), it is incredibly rare that pleasurable anal sex just "happens" with no homework. If you're new to it and want to try it, here are some important tips to remember: *Use a lot of lube. Prep by using toys first, beginning with small butt plugs and graduating to bigger sizes. And GO SLOW.* None of this has to happen all in one go, either. Rome wasn't built in a day, you know. And if anal sex isn't for you, no stress! There are so many ways to get off; find what works for you. Regardless, if you are nervous about trying any new sexual act—and in order to maximize your enjoyment of said act—it is essential to talk through your desires and concerns.

Phew. Are you feeling a little more comfortable with opening up dialogue to expand your sexual consciousness? Now let's apply the same philosophy to the topics that tend to wreak havoc on a relationship, such as finances, children, or affairs. We may fear we don't (yet) have the skills to move forward in our communication about these more complicated subjects without resentment or resistance. However, if each partner takes responsibility for their side of the conversation, we can all learn the skills to hear what really goes on with each other internally.

Are you in the first year (or two or three) of raising kids and having zero to very little sex? Are you resentful because your partner makes more (or less) money than you and expects more (or does less) at home because of it? What are your boundaries around monogamy when you enter into a sexual relationship? What about a married, live-in, or long-term relationship? Have your feelings around monogamy or sexual tastes changed since you've been together? Do you regularly check in with each other? How do you feel about emotional affairs? Have you consensually adopted a "Don't ask, don't tell" policy? Or have you left all these things unsaid but assume the other person is on the same page as you?

Can you talk about these things aloud, even though it may be difficult? Let's say you are in a monogamous long-term relationship and you want to open it up or are attracted to someone else. Could you voice these feelings to your partner instead of either cheating or avoiding talking about it? The fact is, you will be enchanted by other people in the course of a monogamous relationship. This is human. Remember, we're constantly fighting against a basic instinct to mate with as many people as possible.

It's good to talk in the early phase of falling in love about the possibility of infidelity and what each of your boundaries are around "cheating." For example, what would you consider cheating in that particular relationship? Flirting? Watching porn? Sliding into someone's DMs? Having an emotional affair? What one person thinks infidelity means may not include penetration or even real-life sex. Having these conversations (and updating them regularly throughout your relationship) helps each person understand why certain behaviors may be loaded to their partner. It's not that one behavior (such as watching porn) is categorically "wrong," but ongoing communication allows you to reframe it around what feelings the behavior brings up for you, why it bothers you.

The popular podcast *Call Her Daddy* had a catchphrase, "Cheat or be cheated on," which, although funny, I find especially toxic. Instead of challenging the system ("Hurt someone before they can hurt you"), are we going to accept the status quo even if it is ugly and brings out the worst in human behavior? If you aren't getting your needs met in a partnership, talk about it, for fuck's sake! It is totally normal to have a love attachment to one person and also have lust or romantic attraction toward another. But more often than not, rather than face a partner and express these desires, we try to solve problems on our own, which only leads to distrust. So many people share with me how they regularly go through their significant other's phones, emails, and DMs looking for signs of betrayal *instead of* having open communication around these issues. Imagine all the other things we could be thinking about and doing if we freed ourselves from playing private eye on the sly!

My late mentor, the sex and relationship therapist and professor Dr. Walter Brackelmanns, told me that **"if you suggest anything nice about infidelity . . . it stirs up feelings of right and wrong, American flag, apple pie, justice. . . . Rather than looking at the objective reality of whether there is any value to an affair, [we] tend to treat it like it's evil. It's not a question of if it is right or wrong—is it working for you?"** Walter's technique to deal with an affair in therapy was first to determine why the person having the affair was doing it. Did they need to get caught? Did they want out of the primary relationship? Often the person having an affair doesn't want to split up. They are cheating because there is a problem in the relationship and they can't face it, let alone communicate with their partner.

According to Walter, an affair can sustain or even improve a marriage. He frequently suggested patients send a thank-you note to the "other party" after six months to a year of finding out. Whether the relationship recovers or ends, the affair forces hidden issues onto the table. "**If you add oxygen to an affair—bring it into the open—you run the risk of it ending or it becoming a relationship. An affair is like delicate china, [whereas] a committed partnership is like a goldfish. It can sustain a lot of abuse and survive.**" He said an emotional affair is even "trickier" than a consummated one because it exists "in darkness."

If you and your partner choose to be monogamous and you find yourself in a situation where you're intrigued by someone else and tempted to explore, would you be willing to discuss it openly before any lines are crossed? Together, could you decide what feels right for the relationship and either evolve or affirm your boundaries?

Can we stay *receptive* and listen to each other when we come up against obstacles or our own triggers in a conversation? Effective communication requires *active listening*. It is so hard to check our ego and judgment at the door when someone is telling us something we may not be prepared for, not want to hear, or don't agree with. Is it possible to really attempt to take in what they are saying rather than internally formulating our response or defense? Could we stop and pause for a moment before responding?

Here are some tips for actively listening:

1. When someone is speaking to you about their emotions or an experience, especially if it is a sensitive topic, try to *focus on what they are saying rather than how it makes you feel.*

2. Before you respond, notice the following: Are you in the heat of anger? Hungry? Tired? Are you able to speak without yelling? Do you want to hurt them because what they said hurt you? Do you want to criticize?

3. If any of the above rings true, it is a good idea to pause and collect your thoughts before you answer back. You can even say something to the effect of "Thank you for sharing with me. This is a lot

for me to process, and I need some time to be able to respond thoughtfully." Taking a pause helps us to *readjust before responding*.

4. But taking a pause might seem impossible to do! Especially if the person we are communicating with hits below the belt or if resentments have been building up over a period of time. They may have peed all over the toilet seat, left dirty socks on the floor for you to pick up, and forgotten to take out the garbage, *again*—but is it relevant to the current conversation? Is there a different, kinder way to phrase your frustration? (I know it sucks being the bigger person.)

5. The more you practice pausing and becoming aware or *conscious* of how you communicate, the easier it gets over time. The pause is especially helpful when dealing with text arguments (I cannot engage anymore) or social media trolls (I respond only when I am feeling really feisty).

Our internal critics and judges particularly tend to come out when we listen to others through the sometimes self-righteous lens of our own perspective. I remember Nina Hartley telling me years ago that she found it especially difficult for her and others in the kink community to find a great therapist who would accept them without shaming them or trying to uncover some childhood trauma that had caused them to lead an alternative lifestyle. Walter Brackelmanns was adamant that sex therapists work even harder on their own limitations and sexual judgments if they want to treat patients successfully. We all have biases where we lay what we think is right upon other people.

I've been called diplomatic more than once, perhaps because I try to detach and observe whether my own opinion is getting in the way of me listening to someone else's truth. I might not like what they have to say, but I find that the more calm and objective I stay, the less defensive and angry I am when I open my mouth to speak. I wasn't always like this! When I was nineteen and going to art school in New York, I used to rage at the right-to-lifers picketing outside of the abortion clinic that was in the same building as one of my studio classes. I would furiously scream at the top of my lungs because I believe wholeheartedly in a person's reproductive freedom. But at the end of the day, my spewing hate back in their direction didn't improve my mood, my day, or women's right to a legal abortion.

I decided (much later) to try approaching situations like this with *mindful communication.* For me, it helps to write down all the things I am thinking and feeling in order to collect my thoughts. I try to take a day or two and make sure my outrage, for example, is not directing my response. Recently I had to take time out from a close friendship when it became clear that neither of us was in a place to be able to hear each other regarding a sensitive topic. Sometimes taking a little space allows people to reflect and come back on better terms instead of bringing a whole other set of frustrations and experiences to the table that have nothing to do with what you are discussing. Sometimes you just have to agree to disagree or else evaluate whether a situation or relationship is worth fighting for.

When it comes to the current proliferation of cancel culture, there is a benefit to stopping and thinking before commenting on a situation outside of ourselves. This is the moment to ask ourselves whether our point is landing effectively. From behind the scenes at a sex education company, I can attest that it is usually a lack of education and information that leads to people being judgmental—and often, finding the right language to deliver the message makes all the difference.

Just because we like something or see the world a certain way does not mean that we get to impose that set of beliefs on others. Nor does it necessarily mean that there is something wrong with them or with us if we don't agree. I've often found that in spaces where people are prone to open dialogue around sex or consider themselves to be "woke," they have a tendency to be just as or *even more* judgmental than people who might be labeled "conservative." On our The Sex Ed team group chat, we call them SWSJWs, or "super woke social justice warriors." I have been on the receiving end of their wrath so often online that sometimes I want to throw my phone into the ocean!

I've had countless conversations with queer, sex-positive people who say they don't understand how someone could be asexual (the sexual orientation indicative of those who lack sexual attraction to others and/or deprioritize sex as a means of relating to others). From their vantage point, asexuality is *unthinkable.* I also have to remind so many straight "feminist" women that, yes, straight men have feelings too and are just as vulnerable as they are. You'd be surprised how much miscommunication happens because we are so wrapped up in our own version of reality that we completely fail to see someone else's perspective.

I am 100 percent guilty of the above, by the way. Especially so in the past, when it came to communicating effectively with the men in my life. It is important to me personally (as a woman who loves men) and professionally (as a woman who believes that we have all been stuck perpetuating broken behavioral cycles) to be inclusive and welcoming to men, instead of beating them over the head with a sex-positive feminist stick (which, to be totally honest, I have done for much of my life).

Men are perhaps the most trapped by the patriarchy that governs most global societies. They have been brought up to reject emotional vulnerability, to deny their fear, to express emotions as rage, to devalue love and intimacy in favor of disassociative sex—all because these behaviors are deemed more "masculine."

How do we change these old stories and teach young boys new ways of identifying with themselves, love, and healthy masculinity? Our current patriarchal system isn't working for anyone. How can I, as the founder of a sex-positive site, include straight men in the conversations we are having and make them allies instead of foes?

Right now, men—especially white, heterosexual ones—are questioning their voices and what roles they play culturally, professionally, and sexually in a way they never have before. They have been put in check for the first time on a mass level. Whereas once men's virility was never called into question, now society is telling them that they are impotent. Many men feel dismissed by the current backlash, which creates a feeling of not belonging and a defensiveness. (Hence the proclivity for the "not all men" and "father of girls" disclaimers.) I look around and don't see all that many safe places for men to express themselves at a time when they feel they've lost their voices.

I identify with the collective rage and trauma that surrounds patriarchy, yet I also have a strong desire to help heal the narrative in any way I can.

Growing up in a family of alpha males, I've often felt resentment because I did not get the same opportunities I've seen the men in my life get. This has been complicated by the fact that I love and am sexually attracted to men. I've found myself in competition with them, wanting what they have, but ultimately failing to get it, as there is no competition because the playing field is uneven no matter what—even if I tend to be an alpha woman when it comes to my career. I ended up spending too much time trying to prove myself or gain their respect and, in the process, alienating them. This was me participating in a patriarchal narrative of "Power is good, and I must win or prove myself at all costs." But what exactly is the prize? As I try to evolve away from communicating with men from feelings of unfairness and anger, I find myself constantly needing to check whether I am speaking from a place of defensiveness, taking the offense, or actually moving the dialogue forward in a useful way.

As the sex-positive community grows in both visibility and popularity, I've come across a common gap: men are being excluded from the crucial cultural conversations that are being had in this space. These include conversations about consent, pleasure, desire, and more. Which leads me to think about the ways in which men are being left behind. #MeToo[21] as a noun has entered our lexicon, but a lot of the time, we're not including men in dialogues about how or why sexual harassment and abuse happen, and we are *definitely* not doing enough to listen to them in the aftermath.

Often, straight men will tell me that they fear being judged or "canceled" if they aren't up on the latest nomenclature for gender and sexual identity. They are concerned they are addicted to porn but afraid that if they voice this to their partners they will be shamed. And they want to know more about intimacy, about pleasure, about how to navigate sexual encounters in a post–#MeToo world.

I've come to the conclusion that we need to be creating more spaces for men to be vulnerable, to be nurtured, and to participate in healing from the centuries of wounded masculinity that has kept them in boxes. As bell hooks wrote in *The Will to Change: Men, Masculinity, and Love*, "Men cannot change if there are no blueprints for change. Men cannot love if they are not taught the art of loving."

I want men to be part of a new paradigm of sexual pleasure. To help men come into their own divine masculinity and feel uplifted and supported as they unpack the nuances of an entirely new frontier of sexuality and gender politics. Selfishly, I want to improve my relationships with men, too. Much of this boils down to creating healthier discourse all around.

In every single case I've outlined above, being clear on our own feelings, stating them aloud clearly, and consciously listening to others only help to improve communication and relationships. When we confront things we might normally avoid, they have less power over us. And the more explicit we are about our expectations and boundaries around sex and love, the more fulfilling they can be.

---

21 Conceived in 2006 by survivor and advocate Tarana Burke, a little over a decade later this sociopolitical initiative aimed at breaking silence surrounding sex-related traumas would ramp up its visibility via Twitter and Instagram hashtags. Unprecedented numbers of high-profile individuals speaking candidly about their experiences culminated in one of the culture's most significant contemporary paradigm shifts; many assert that in 2017, the mainstream media's attitude toward survivors of sexual abuse, assault, and harassment pivoted from one of de facto skepticism and/or blame to one of belief and affirmation for truth telling.

To recap, mindful communication—and this goes across the board, from romantic and sexual relationships to family dynamics—requires:

1. Identifying and honestly expressing your own wants, needs, and feelings, even when it may be uncomfortable or awkward to do so.

2. Practicing active listening and not planning your response while someone is speaking. Try to stay neutral and objective, and notice if some of your old wounds are being triggered, such as abandonment, rejection, or resentment.

3. Risking receiving a response you may not like in exchange for the potential of greater pleasure.

It sounds simple when typed out in a straightforward list, but the struggle to stay mindful in the moment is real. The more we train ourselves to *slow down* and listen (to ourselves and others), the easier it is to do. I promise.

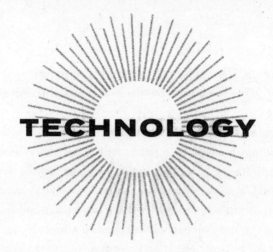

TECHNOLOGY

Humans are wired to seek out other human beings for love, companionship, romance, sex. We have a primal desire to mate, whether or not our intention is to produce offspring. We differ from primates in that we also desire emotional, mental, spiritual, and physical intimacy.

While we may be driven to have closeness with one another, we spend most of our time actively avoiding empathetic, vulnerable exchanges. Technology plays a big role in how and why we have become so disconnected from our *humanity*. Digital connectivity, while liberating and democratizing, has also led us to have less empathy, less intimacy, and less emotional intelligence.

We now inhabit a consistent half-present, half-distracted state as we multitask between our virtual world and our actual existence. Have you ever been on your phone in the checkout line at the grocery store, texting or having a conversation while the cashier rings up your purchases? What about while waiting for someone at a bar, restaurant, movie theater, or club? Do you reach for your device to fill up those awkward pauses instead of looking around at people, catching their eye, striking up a conversation with a stranger, or—the horror—sitting alone in silent observation wherever it is you happen to be? It's more common than not for us to be on our phones while having an IRL experience solo or with others—at dinner, in a meeting, in bed, taking a walk, even while driving.

Sometimes, to force myself to be fully present, I'll leave my phone at home when I go out. It doesn't take long before I find myself fidgeting, reflexively reaching for my device. I get uncomfortable, as I'm often the only one not looking down at a screen. I feel like not looking at my phone makes me seem like I'm not normal. The void begins to fill me with insecurity and anxiety, and I am reminded of how far away from being at peace with one another and the in-between moments we have become.

Earlier in this book, I talked about the *void* and our impulsive need to fill it. Well, technology is a tool for instant gratification and validation that most of us now share. It's hard to believe there was even a time when we had to practice social skills on a daily basis. A time when we were forced to exchange basic pleasantries with other people, when it was considered rude not to look someone in the eye and experience them as a real human being. Can you even imagine that people used to send and receive love letters (I still do—call me old-fashioned) and wait, sometimes for weeks, when mail was carried by ships for a response? Now, if we miss someone or we feel a little lonely or sad, we can send out messages to a vast number of contacts and wait for someone to reply back and confirm that we are valued.

Technology is a double-edged sword. On the one hand, it's an amazing tool that has given us so many ways of reaching people across the globe who mirror our experiences. Up through the early 2000s, someone struggling with sexual and gender identity may have felt totally alienated in their corner of the world. Now we have the opportunity to find community and acceptance in a hand-held device, even if we can't find it at home.

As cyberspace bridges us together, it is also cutting us off from community, nature (if you've ever Instagrammed a sunset, you know what I mean), and true bonding with one another. Our screens act as a sort of self-defense. We hide behind them; they give us courage to say and do things we may not ever conceive of admitting IRL. On social media we may be exposing the depths of our souls—sharing journeys of mental health, traumas, sexual orientation, body image, and other vulnerable subjects—with complete strangers. Yet it seems unthinkable to tell a stranger in real life a quarter of what we reveal on-line. Somehow it is less tender to reveal our experiences and feelings virtually.

We may find ourselves turning to social media to feel affirmation when we are at our lowest, needing to share our grief, wanting to commemorate or celebrate our joy. Humans used to prove existence by carving their names into a tree or rock. Now we can post a pic to prove that we were there, we are valid, and we are worthy of your "likes." Holidays can be an especially triggering time on social media. I recall feeling an invisible pressure to post a picture of my dad on Father's Day because everyone else in my feed was, even though (1) he's dead, so (2) he wouldn't see my post. I intellectually understand that I'm ridiculous for playing into the mentality of "If I don't post, do I exist?" and I could just take the space off-line to feel the loss—but damn, FOMO (fear of missing out) is real!

It's disheartening to witness how many people all around the world are struggling with being vulnerable and intimate, particularly in romantic and/or sexual relationships. Truly *seeing* other people and allowing yourself to be *seen* can be scary. I frequently hear how self-conscious people feel when someone looks them in the eye during (generally casual) sex—a truly intimate act.

In the twenty-first century, sex and love have moved online—easy to come by, dispensable. There are a plethora of options at our fingertips, vast menus of hookup and dating apps categorized by gender, sexual, and even financial preference. It's never been easier to find other humans with whom to couple (or thruple). With endless choices, we can continually refresh, trade up, and consider all our options instead of committing to someone we may eventually tire of. There's a dopamine hit from text flirtation, someone exciting sliding into our DMs, liking and commenting on every post without the commitment of an actual relationship. It's indicative of our half-present, half-distracted digital mating habits. Interestingly, recent studies have shown that millennials and Gen Z'ers are having less sex (including less casual sex) than ever before—in part due to the amount of time they spend scrolling.

With all the progress global interconnectivity offers, culturally we are slipping further away from kinship. As we live more of our existence virtually, how can we merge the innovations of technology with humanity and greater consciousness?

Sherry Turkle is a professor in the Program in Science, Technology, and Society at MIT and the founding director of the MIT Initiative on Technology and Self. With a PhD in sociology and personality psychology, Turkle does work centered on the study of how humans interact with technology. In 2012, she presented a TED Talk (since translated into more than thirty languages) that proposed a crucial question: Are we "connected, but alone?" "Technology appeals to us most where we are most vulnerable," she says in the talk.

> And we are vulnerable. We're lonely, but we're afraid of intimacy. And so from social networks to sociable robots, we're designing technologies that will give us the illusion of companionship without the demands of friendship. We turn to technology to help us feel connected in ways we can comfortably control. But we're not so comfortable. We are not so much in control. These days, those phones in our pockets are changing

> our minds and hearts because they offer us three gratifying fantasies. One,
> that we can put our attention wherever we want it to be; two, that we
> will always be heard; and three, that we will never have to be alone. And
> that third idea, that we will never have to be alone, is central to changing
> our psyches. Because the moment that people are alone, even for a few
> seconds, they become anxious, they panic, they fidget, they reach for a
> device. . . . Being alone feels like a problem that needs to be solved.

Speaking of being alone and the human condition of needing other humans: technology has helped us hack the "problem" of meeting a mate. Dating and hookup apps are a multi-billion-dollar industry. Their algorithms promise to deliver love, sex, a financial arrangement—the perfect match. But they also induce social awkwardness and further disengagement from intimacy. The more reliant we are on machines to facilitate our emotional, romantic, and sexual partnerships, the less intelligent we become in these areas.

I'll often go through friends' messaging services on various dating apps (with their invitation and consent) to see how they digitally communicate with potential partners. It's common on heteronormative apps for people to carry on endless text dialogue (I'm talking paragraphs exchanged over a number of days or weeks) without meeting up IRL. I've seen many cases of emotional devastation by a virtual "relationship" ending even with little to no face-to-face time involved. I've seen heterosexual men position themselves as emotionally available and nurturing by copying and pasting a standard message such as "I'm at Whole Foods, want anything?" to a string of prospective mates. These kinds of behaviors create a false sense of intimacy. Establishing true intimacy takes time—and emotional risk. When we rush a connection, furiously exchanging messages back and forth, we avoid the uncertainty that comes with getting to know someone authentically.

People often complain about using dating apps and wish they could meet someone in the course of regular life. Have humans suddenly changed so radically since we got handheld devices that the randomness of finding a romantic spark through locking eyes or speaking to a stranger has disappeared? Or have we just become too uncomfortable to look up from our phones and engage in conversation?

We live in a culture in which we use technology to interact with each other without having learned how to treat each other with genuine decency online. Our deficit of literacy regarding empathy, subtlety, and even basic politeness in cyberspace often shows up as extreme boundary crossing when it comes to engaging romantically. For example, let's say someone doesn't match with a person they're after on an app. Instead of leaving it be, many will seek out their unrequited crush on social media and slide into the DMs there. Okay, chill. If they didn't want to date you on one platform, take it as a hard no regarding reaching out to them elsewhere. At The Sex Ed, we get so many questions about dating apps, ghosting, and dick pics that sometimes I think I should write a sex etiquette manual for the digital age.

Let's talk about ghosting.[22] This is indicative of the type of passive-aggressive communication I mentioned in the last chapter. If we are physically intimate enough with someone to exchange any kind of bodily fluids, we should be able to say to them, "I think you're great, but not for me" or "I don't think either of us needs to spend more time together" instead of engaging in digital silence. The person may be really into us (or us into them), but that doesn't mean the feeling is reciprocated. Not acknowledging a lack of interest when someone follows up for more contact is downright rude. Unless you are dealing with a stalker, psychopath, or someone who won't take no for an answer, honesty is usually the best policy.

Regarding the sending and receiving of nudes, if you are lucky enough to receive them, do you understand that the (generally unstated) understanding is that they are for your eyes only? Do you share them with your friends? Or, worse, post them online?

Comedian Joel Kim Booster experienced his nudes being leaked online and strangers commenting on his dick size. He told me,

> They ended up on one message board. The reviews are good,
> nobody's shitty about them. Yet all these strangers on the Internet
> were picking apart my dick pics. It's interesting to read. Sometimes
> people will be like, "This is gross." And then the automatic response
> is, "Well, if they didn't want the pictures shown, they shouldn't have
> taken them." This is how far down the rabbit hole of that thinking
> you can go before you can justify anything. Then, on the other hand,

---

22 A passive-aggressive form of digital dating nonetiquette, this is the phenomenon of abruptly ceasing communication. The strategy is often employed by those who are uncomfortable with direct communication and setting clear boundaries; they therefore seek to forgo the complications and obligations of further communication. Reasons range from fear of communicating directly to discomfort with the establishment of boundaries, but one thing's for sure: if you've been ghosted, you probably shouldn't hold your breath waiting for an answer.

I'm not ashamed of my body. That being said, I would love for them to be taken down just because I would like to have some semblance of control over who sees my body. But at the end of the day, I think my generation especially, [our intimate images] are all going to get out there eventually, and to waste too much emotional energy about it is probably just going to cause me to spiral.

For most people raised on digital devices and porn, it is a rite of passage to sext and exchange nudes.[23] You can't tell people not to do so, but we can educate people on how to respect boundaries around sharing intimate photos. We should not have to assume a risk that if we send a lover a nude, maybe one day it could end up in public.

Carrie Goldberg is a victims' rights attorney and founder of C. A. Goldberg, a cutting-edge law firm that helps victims fight "psychos, stalkers, pervs, and trolls," with prominent cases against the New York Department of Education and Grindr. Carrie's own experience with a vengeful ex changed the course of her career, which she details in her book *Nobody's Victim*. As she says,

Millennials have been raised with their cell phone not just within arm's reach but attached to their hand, and have grown up using the Internet and their phones for everything. There's nothing we don't use the Internet to do. Of course it's going to expand to include sexuality and dating and be a tool for that. I certainly think that it's unrealistic to say, "Don't take the pictures in the first place." But we should say, "If you are entrusted with intimate pictures of somebody else, don't share those." I mean, that's where the emphasis is. Certain information should be treated as private. We accept that credit card numbers and social security numbers are private information, and we would be a lot less humiliated if those got leaked. . . . We are a lot less humiliated when somebody tries to use our credit card, and yet that's criminal behavior.

---

23   "Send nudes," "n00dz?," or any other queries involving this word typically are a sign that the sender is requesting photos in which the receiver is naked. When you're sending nudes, be sure to let the person know the photo is for their eyes only (if that is your intention), and be sure to keep any identifying physical attributes out of the photos (such as your face or tattoos) to protect your anonymity should these photos be shared without your consent. If you're a recipient of nudes, you are very lucky, so treat them with the respect you'd give a piece of fine art!

A note (especially to hetero men) regarding dick pics: please don't send unsolicited ones; only send if they've been explicitly requested. Some people love a dick pic; I have many friends who have hundreds saved on their phones, images they specifically sought out. Yet most women receive so many unwelcome ones, frequently from complete strangers—my unread DM requests on any given day contain an abundance. My friend the adult superstar Riley Reid, whose videos have been viewed more than a billion times on PornHub, has a genius operation for dick pics. On her OnlyFans account, she charges subscribers for her to rate their dicks. It's only a few bucks per message, but when you consider that she receives hundreds to thousands of photo requests per week, it adds up. Maybe we should all start charging.

Social media specializes in triggering us to perform idealized versions of ourselves, our sexuality, even our committed and romantic partnerships (as in making it "Instagram official"). The norm is filters and Facetune, Kardashian-esque curves and hard bodies presented in an endless scroll of selfies. When I consider what kids who grew up with smartphones have to contend with and deprogram as "normal"—now that social media has upended, heightened, and entirely fucked with our ideas of "normal" to the billionth degree—I shudder. Normal is now so unrealistic and unattainable that teenagers feel pressure to submit to plastic surgery and injectables to reach an ever-higher bar. That translates to expressing their sexuality for acceptance in even higher degrees. TikTok is inundated with eleven-year-olds executing perfect WAP[24] choreography before they can understand what effect their bodies performing these moves might have on others' desires.

Much of our performative use of technology has been influenced by streaming porn. It's no surprise, considering that adult webmasters learned to monetize the Internet faster than anyone else. There would be no gamers, YouTubers, TikTokkers, or celebrities capitalizing on their followers if porn stars and producers hadn't done it first.

Full disclosure: I do not think that pornography is evil and should be stopped or avoided at all costs. I think we need to be able, as a society, to engage critically with an industry that belongs to one of the oldest professions: sex work. Unlike any

---

24 This acronym for "wet-ass pussy" is the title of a 2020 chart-topping hip-hop single recorded by Cardi B and Megan Thee Stallion. The single serves as an anthem for many, eroticizing the singers' vaginal anatomy in (among a host of other innuendo- and pun-laden phrases) a celebratory likening of its moisture to that of "macaroni in a pot."

other kind of sex work, pornography exists at the nexus of media, entertainment, and technology. It has become ingrained in all these aspects of our lives, whether we like it or not. The amplification these "legitimate" industries lend to porn has made it a beast that can tame us into submission, unless we learn to understand how it affects our cultural and personal relationships to sexuality.

During the second wave of feminism (the 1960s through early 1990s), many in the movement were vehemently antiporn, actively denigrating women who worked in the adult industry instead of including them in the struggle for equal rights. (Yet another example of white feminism's failure to be intersectional.)[25] Unfortunately, scores of "enlightened" people still adopt a blanket ideology of "Porn is bad and treats women like sex objects and is immoral." It's not that simple.

Porn can be a useful tool for exploring personal sexuality and bringing passion back into relationships, *and* it can also lead to numerous insecurities and bad habits. Many sex therapists will suggest clients watch specific adult content as a way to open up their sexual preferences and expand their pleasure solo or in a partnership. If we aren't getting the modeling or healthy sex education anywhere else, what other options do we have? Pornography is how most of the planet is now learning about sex. Where else can you see clear depictions of vulvas, penises, blow jobs, anal sex, or even plain ol' missionary?

Contemporary sex education must include porn literacy. This means learning the skills to interpret what we see, question how we interact with porn, and gain more consciousness about how we absorb adult content *mindfully*. We need to be having emotional and psychological conversations in order to process the information we are taking in.

Porn has been around since the dawn of time and isn't going anywhere. I'm not saying I love the current landscape of the adult business and streaming sites (in terms of both available mainstream content and who benefits economically on the back end) or that it is largely ethical or inclusive, but hey, neither is Hollywood.

Back in the day, prior to home streaming and personal computers, it was really difficult to access X-rated materials. You had to go to a sex shop to buy a

---

25 This term refers to contemporary culture's acknowledgment of the individual's ability to claim multiple identities. Here, for example, a person may assert (among endless potential core identities) their racial background, disability, and/or sobriety while also doing so in regard to their immigration, HIV, and/or domestic-abuse-survivor statuses. Queer people of color are perhaps one of the most media-visible examples of a hybrid space of identity. Ultimately these efforts to create new language aim to carve our restorative spaces of acknowledgment for many whose experiences have been previously overshadowed or ignored.

"dirty" magazine or rent a porn movie on VHS. A salesperson would generally wrap the item in a brown paper bag. Consuming adult material was a discreet and taboo process. Even further back in time, you'd have to order your porn from the back of a mail-order catalog and enclose a self-addressed stamped envelope. Now it's easier than ordering an Uber. Not to mention porn is now divided into so many subgenres (choking, spitting, *bukkake*,[26] *hentai*,[27] gang bang,[28] DP,[29] et cetera, et cetera, etc.); these didn't number in the thousands prior to the advent of streaming smut.

Many spend as much time mindlessly scrolling through streaming porn as they do on Netflix or Instagram. We've become so reliant on visual porn to masturbate that we are raising entire generations who can't get off without it.[30] Moreover, the more we consume and are dependent on a specific type of stimulation to get off, the more our need increases for specialized or hardcore material to acheive arousal.

Joseph Gordon-Levitt wrote, directed, and starred in the 2013 film *Don Jon*, in which his character has an incredibly active sex life but can find sexual gratification only by jacking off to porn. The movie finds him grappling with his porn-viewing habits and his inability to be intimate with women IRL. I wish this film was required sex-ed viewing in high schools! I would say 80 percent of the concerns that straight men under forty express to me are related to their relationship with porn and intimacy.

---

26 If the traditional blow job is a single serving, welcome to an all-you-can-eat buffet. Believed to have been codified in 1980s Japanese porn, this act places a consensual oral "bottom" on the receiving end of multiple ejaculations upon their face.

27 This term is utilized throughout the globe to describe Japanese erotic cartoons, or anime/manga porn. Beyond being merely suggestive, the genre is differentiated by its consistent nudity and thorough depictions of intimate acts. For many, it allows a nonthreatening, fantasy exploration of situations and sex that they might not ever personally venture to experience. Evidence of this is the high percentage of cisgender, heterosexually identifying women who enjoy the genre's gay cis-male-themed niche.

28 A sexual act that involves multiple people (most often) penetrating a single person simultaneously or one at a time.

29 "Double penetration," or the act of penetrating (or being penetrated in) two orifices, such as vagina and anus or anus and mouth. While a person can achieve this layered stimulation with multiple partners, they are not necessary. With enough imagination, lube, and toys, a single partner isn't necessary either. Just be sure that if you have a vagina and you're having fun with anal play, thoroughly clean all fingers and toys before inserting what had been in your anus into your vagina!

30 A note here about the fallacy of "porn addiction." Although the reliance on porn can be categorized within a greater pathology, like sex addiction (another clinical behavioral type that is up for debate by experts), there is currently not enough hard science and research-driven data to back up this theory. Still, oversaturation and use of pornography can absolutely have a detrimental effect on sexual development, response, and behavior.

One successful actor friend of mine, who prefers to remain anonymous (he's a heartthrob with social media followers in the millions), sent me a series of voice notes detailing his complicated alliance with porn. He took pride in sharing that, in an effort to become more conscious about how often he used sexually explicit material to get off, he installed a tracking app on his devices to monitor his smut habit. As I type these words, he has gone without streaming porn for two years, four months, one day, nine hours, five minutes, and sixteen seconds. Could you go a week or a month just to see what happens?

Here's a simple exercise for becoming more intentional about how you consume porn. Try masturbating or becoming aroused using a different kind of stimuli than your usual go-to. For example, if you always watch streaming porn, use still images, audio erotica, a new toy, or even . . . your own imagination. Is it taking you longer to become wet or erect? Do you find yourself frustrated because it is more difficult to get off? Notice these feelings and also ask yourself why you might be rushing through the experience of orgasming—something that is meant to bring you *pleasure and release.*

Recent clinical research shows erectile dysfunction[31] in sexually active men under forty (and even in teenagers) significantly spiked upward after the first streaming porn sites launched around 2006. Low sexual desire and sexual difficulty are also on the rise. Not to mention body image dysmorphia and expectations around pleasure and performance. As sexpert Tyomi Morgan explains,

> When it comes to sex in general, most people are used to the idea
> of performing. I think it comes from the consumption of porn. The
> media feeds into this trope as well in referencing sexual engagement
> as a performance. A lot of times people come to sexual experiences
> with an idea of what sex is supposed to look like, then they feel
> that they have to perform, especially if what their ideas around
> sex looking like involves things that they don't normally gravitate
> toward or techniques that they aren't really good at. They feel like
> they have to put on another personality and pretend and kind of

---

31 This is the inability to obtain or sustain an erection. It can be experienced by those with a penis for a host of reasons, including (but not limited to) stress, substance abuse, and performance anxiety. Studies estimate that this phenomenon's prevalence ranges from 9 to 40 percent among men ages forty and younger, generally increasing by 10 percent with each decade afterward. Though aging appears to be a key factor, many younger individuals navigate, manage, and ultimately address erection challenges throughout their sex lives.

just fuck [their way] through it, or [they're] showing up to put on
the theatrics. I find that people with vulvas or vaginas, especially if
they're not enjoying it, feel like they still have to moan, they still
have to put on the face and do all the extra theatrics for the sake of
feeding into their partner's pleasure.

It's normal to have a complicated association between our sexuality and pornography or compare ourselves to what we see on-screen and to what kind of
porn our partner likes, even though—and especially—because none of it is
real. *Compare and despair*, baby! I get questions like these all the time: "I'm a
heterosexual female in my twenties with a heterosexual male partner. I know
I shouldn't be, but I am hurt knowing he is watching other women in porn.
Something in me *still* feels like I'm not good enough and that is why he is
watching other women. Is there a way to make it feel okay? I'm just so con-
fused, and I'm hoping to hear your take if there are others feeling the same way."

There are countless intelligent, articulate, and perceptive adult stars who
should be fielding these queries instead of me. Why wouldn't we want to take
advice from someone who has more than ten thousand hours in the field? I remember that when I was a kid and DARE (Drug Abuse Resistance Education)
was part of our elementary school curriculum, recovering drug addicts would
come and speak to class. Adult star Jessica Drake is a certified sex educator with
a popular series of ethical instructional adult films on everything from fellatio to
anal sex to basic positions, but I doubt your local high school would have her in
for a lecture. We have plenty of mainstream celebrities telling us why we should
care about climate change or Indigenous rights, even though they may have very
little direct experience in the subject. Yet the performers who have become our
de facto sexual role models—the same ones who may have taught you or your
kids what a blow job looks like—are shut out of the sex-ed dialogue.

Lexington Steele is one of the most well-known male adult film stars in the
world. He is an AVN Hall of Fame porn star with three AVN Performer of the Year
awards. He even has dildos modeled after his own likeness, ones that are admittedly
difficult for the average person to measure themselves against. His advice:

Do not compare yourself to what you see. Do you think that you
could go on the highway and drive the same as a NASCAR driver?
A NASCAR driver could probably drive a hundred miles an hour
in the opposite direction on a major highway and never get in an

accident because they are highly skilled at what they do. The people that do adult movies are highly skilled in what they do, so don't fault yourself for premature ejaculation or underperforming based on performance anxiety. Don't compare yourself to the people that are performing in the movies that you watch. There's a reason the guys that are in this business are built like this and can do this. We're not doing any tricks, but there's a lot of mental gymnastics that are going on in male performers' heads. We didn't just wake up and be like, "I can get my dick hard!" You bomb, and you live to tell about it. One thing about being a male performer is you have to have a short memory and/or a comfort with the memory of underperforming.

Riley Reid, who beyond her entrepreneurial success in the adult space also has numerous adult awards under her belt, notes that

> porn is not sex education. Porn doesn't show the behind-the-scenes of the before and after of us communicating, "What are you okay with? What are you consenting to?" Porn can be very male dominating and the woman acting almost as if maybe she's not enjoying it or [as if] she is enjoying it. We are performance actors. I think it's important to express to people that it's okay to have your fetishes and your sexuality. But the main importance is to explain what consent is and communication. I think communication is something that we don't express enough about. And I think people are just too scared, and so if you force people into these awkward conversations, it helps them learn how to become better at it.

Asa Akira can speak from more than one perspective, as she is not only a renowned porn star but also a mother. Since having children, Asa has been wondering things like

> Wow, what are their first porno experiences going to be? Personally, I love rough sex. And a lot of the porn I've done and shot over the course of my career has been really rough sex. I love gang bangs. I love getting choked. I love getting slapped. And of course, nobody gets to see the behind-the-scenes of that where we have the conversation before the shoot. What I want to do, what I'm into,

what they're into. I don't think the problem is with the porn that we're shooting. I think it's great that we show the whole spectrum of sexuality. If we had better sex ed, I don't think people would look to porn to learn about sex. The ten-year-old boy that has already learned about sex and consent and [that] different people have different tastes—just like in food, or movies, or anything else—I think that's the kid that's not necessarily going to look at gang bang porn and think that is what all sex should look [like]. I think we as a society need to do better with sex ed rather than pointing our fingers at porn and being like, "We shouldn't show that kind of porn." Because those are sexual fantasies that really exist, and I think it's good to normalize all kinds of sex.

Peggy Orenstein is the author of the groundbreaking *New York Times* bestsellers *Girls & Sex* and its follow-up, *Boys & Sex*. As she puts it,

We can talk about feminist porn or ethical porn . . . but that stuff is all behind a paywall. And what is easily accessible to young people and what they're accessing from a really young age is a lot of porn that reinforces that idea that sex is something men do to women and that female pleasure is a performance for male satisfaction. And they are using that because we don't talk to them either about sex or about porn and what's real and what's not real and what's missing and what could or should be. They use [porn] as sex ed.

Of course we want to protect children from growing up too fast and becoming hypersexualized, but the sad reality is that close to 90 percent of children aged eight to fifteen have accidentally or purposefully viewed online porn. This is while most adults are avoiding having basic conversations about sex with their kids until it is "age appropriate." But what is age appropriate these days? I am certainly not suggesting that you tell your seven-year-old about anal sex. I do believe, however, that age-appropriate conversations about sexuality, consent, genitals, and more should happen as soon as your child starts exploring their body and asking you questions. Most of our own discomfort about speaking to our kids about sex comes from us not having done the work ourselves.

But if you've read this far, you're already committed to confronting your own shame around sex and don't want to pass the ancestral trauma and patterns down to a new generation, right? Congrats! You've got the opportunity to raise a healthy, well-adjusted, mindful kid who is going to grow up loving themselves, honoring their body, and having respect for their own and others' boundaries.

As porn has evolved from VHS tapes in paper bags to one-click access, it's easy to see how adult content now dictates so much about how we see ourselves, how we get aroused, and what we expect from a sexual encounter. So how do we evolve to have a better relationship with porn? Porn literacy is the first step. Meaning, having the skills to process and understand our individual and collective relationship to pornography. We make conscious decisions regarding the food and mainstream media we consume but tend to forget this value system when it comes to the porn we watch. For example, because I'm oversaturated with reading, studying, and talking about sex all day, I don't consume porn in my personal life. (Although I do possess a collection of vintage erotica.)

A tipping point for me came in 2012, when I attended the AVN convention and awards show in Las Vegas. In a peculiar twist, I had an offer to be flown to Vegas as a guest of the fashion brand Chanel to attend a series of events for a new store they were opening in the Wynn Las Vegas. When I found out the timing intersected with AVN, you better believe I had my convention passes booked faster than you could say, "It's Chanel, baby!"

As a sex researcher, I approach a convention that's based on pornography to gather consumer data and see the latest product developments, much in the same way I would a car trade show or a fashion trade show. I'm there to find out things like what the top-selling dildos are, how much market share they have, what their customer makeup is, and who is the top-grossing adult star. My porn is analytics. Consider the fact that a streaming adult site like PornHub has 100 million page views a day. It is as recognizable as a mainstream media or luxury brand like HBO or Chanel, with a higher Q score (a measure of consumer familiarity with a brand) and possibly more influence on culture.

My boyfriend at the time tagged along and was completely repulsed, overwhelmed, and a bit distressed at this peek behind the curtain. I remember him saying to me, incredulously, "But it's not sexy!" That night, the rapper Too $hort was performing at the end of the awards show, and we wanted to stick around long enough to see him, but the list of nominee categories was like a thick dictionary. Whereas in the heyday of Paul Fishbein, creator of the awards show, there may have been fourteen or fifteen categories, by 2012, with endless subgenres to be recognized, the show was stretching longer than the Academy Awards. Even the masses of flesh on display couldn't hold our attention long enough for us to make it through. We were both so wiped out from a full day of interacting with sexual content that we likely passed out without having any that night.

Part of the problem is that most porn comes across as routine and soulless. As Nina Hartley observes, "In our culture, if you make sex art, it's called pornography because we don't value sexuality enough to let the great artists handle it. But sex and passion and pleasure are equally as worthy of artistic endeavor as love and death and war and allegory and the Bible. Each culture gets the pornography it deserves because the explicit material we put on screen is a reflection of culture, not an engine of culture."

If it's true we have the pornography our culture deserves, then it would seem to be that we (mostly) see sex as rote, unfeeling, devoid of intimacy. "I think our attention spans and our diffusion of emotion, whether it be toward porn or toward the phone, hasn't really been dug into," actor Ramy Youssef told me. "**I think about the access that my friends and I had with porn at such an early age. In my show [*Ramy*], my character talks about watching more porn in order to not have sex. I think that's something that's very real to me, and understanding that there's a difference between what happens in porn and what real intimacy is.**"

On a personal level, we need to be more tuned in to the ways we may be using pornography to avoid our void or intimacy with others. On a collective level, we should question how intertwined our sexuality is with technology. Gray Scott, a futurist, techno-philosopher, and one of the world's leading experts in the field of emerging technology, points out that "we have been in a sexual relationship with machines for a very long time, whether it was a VHS tape recorder with a porn [video] on it or an iPhone that you're masturbating to a video on. So you're already in a sexual encounter with a machine, and with smartphones, we've already migrated into the sexual experience including an AI that's in the room with you."

This is the kind of stuff that sends me down rabbit holes, wondering whether—for all the myriad ways tech has improved our lives—it is also having a devastating effect on our sense of intimacy, love, and consciousness in the present and in the future. Has technology divorced us from romantic and sexual intimacy to such an extent that there's no turning back? Or is there a possibility of engaging with technology and even developing new forms of it that might help us be connected and together instead of connected and alone? What if we instituted new forms of digital etiquette when it comes to love, sex, and online relationships? Could we make it a regular practice to unplug from our devices? I wonder what kind of unexpected human connections we might make if we put the phone away the next time we were at dinner or in the checkout line and we tuned in to the reality right in front of us.

I believe that to be awakened to our digital reality and how it affects our sexual desires, experiences, and relationships means becoming conscious about our relationship with technology. That might mean applying your own critical thinking and research as more and more misinformation is spread online as gospel (even and especially within your own algorithmic bubble), or considering how your digital life heightens your sense of *compare and despair*, or setting limits on your leisure-time technology use. One way I enact a limit for myself is by doing periodic detoxes from social media, for example, by taking Friday through Monday morning off Instagram. It often makes me laugh at myself to see how long I can or cannot go without checking the feed. But when I do take time off, I notice I feel a lot less FOMO and a lot more clear. It is a virtual world, after all, not our immediate environment. Because technology has taken over most of our interactions, there is more need than ever to become conscious of our surroundings, our communities, and the sweet, sexy, nurturing relationships we may notice and have time for if and when we become *present*.

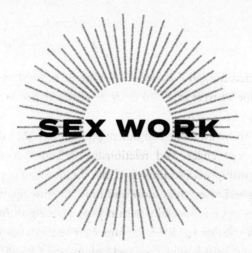

SEX WORK

Trigger warning: This chapter details a topic that many people find disturbing, which is prostitution, now more often referred to as "sex work." Before we get into how to have sacred sex and enjoy the transcendent intuitive wisdom of our bodies, which will be covered in the second half of this book, I want to talk about this subject, one that most people would rather ignore. I mentioned earlier, when talking about filling the void, the concept of spiritual bypassing, or ignoring our shadows. I find that often in the self-help and New Age circles, *there is a tendency to be in a "good vibes only" bubble* that doesn't acknowledge the collective healing we need around the darker side of humanity when it comes to sex.

I am all for love and light and expanding pleasure, or I wouldn't have written this book. However, I believe that being *conscious about sex* and the outdated system we have all been operating within (our old normal) includes understanding *the economy around sex*. So in order to say "Fuck the system"and build a new one, we are going to have to talk about sex work.

Because sex is a basic human need, there has always existed an economy around it. Reliable and recent statistics on the percentages of people who pay for sex are hard to come by, because of the high stigma and dearth of research around the subject. Various studies conducted in the twenty-first century estimate around 15 to 20 percent of Americans have visited a sex worker. Numbers vary per country, with Italy, Spain, and Japan hovering around 30 to 45 percent and places where sex work is legalized trending higher—for example, Cambodia and Thailand, at 59 to 80 percent. Chances are, you or someone in your close circle has at some point exchanged money for some kind of sexual service, even if it was a "massage with release." Whatever your personal experience or moral compass is around sex work, it exists, it isn't going anywhere, and it is a component in our understanding of the human psyche and experience of sex. *If reading about it isn't for you, please feel free to skip this chapter. If you decide to keep reading, I ask for your consciousness and compassion as we approach this fraught topic.*

Whether regulated or criminalized, revered or reviled, sex work has origins in almost every single civilization on the planet. In many (if not all) countries around the world colonized by Europeans, women were regularly claimed as "prizes" or sold into sexual slavery by colonizers; bodily autonomy and rights they had were stripped away. The world has not been just to those born with a vagina between their legs.

The ancient Roman city of Pompeii, which was sealed off by the eruption of Mount Vesuvius in AD 79, has a preserved brothel district that you can still visit. Here you'll find giant phalluses on the exterior doorways indicating what kind of business existed within and erotic paintings on the inside walls depicting services offered. Present-day archaeologists and historians estimate that one of every five workers in these brothels (male and female) were enslaved.

Have you ever heard the expression "worth your weight in gold"? This phrase originated during the California gold rush of the late 1840s, when miners, alongside pioneer female sex workers, settled the Wild West. Before proper saloons could be built, makeshift drinking tents were set up. On a bar made from wooden planks, there would be a double-sided scale. Now mind you, this is the early days of the rush, and gold currency wasn't yet fixed. After a long day of mining, the men would place gold nuggets on one side of the scale, and their choice of woman would stand on the other. When the scales were even, the price for the night was settled, hence "worth your weight in gold." The vogue back then for women's figures was referred to as "beef stock," implying a heftier build, which in turn led to a heftier profit for the brothel.

Flash-forward a hundred-plus years, and at the upper echelon of sex work we find famous twentieth-century madams like Heidi Fleiss, who serviced Hollywood; Sydney Biddle Barrows, "the Mayflower Madam," who catered to East Coast elite; and Madame Claude in Paris, who booked women for high-profile clients from the 1960s to the '80s throughout Europe, the US, and the Middle East.

When it comes to lower-priced options, there's the famed Bois de Boulogne in Paris, a location with a long history of street-level sex workers, or Hollywood Boulevard in Los Angeles, the backdrop for Sean Baker's brilliant 2015 film

Tangerine, about transgender sex workers, and also the area where movie star Hugh Grant was arrested for soliciting sex from Divine Brown in 1995.

No matter how much culture, technology, economics, or legal issues have changed over the centuries, there have been very few improvements to or understanding of this industry and its reach.

Let's break it down.

Sex work is the consensual exchange of sexual services for money or goods (which can include food, shelter, luxury items, or basic necessities). Sexual services can stretch beyond sex acts to include emotional labor, such as building self-esteem, creating an illusion of love, or providing intimacy, companionship, and comfort. Sometimes these services include tending to various kinks, accommodating physical conditions (for example, working with disabled clients who may have difficulty finding willing partners), or being on the receiving end of degrading acts. Sex workers (SWs for short) ply their trade with others, individually, or for another person or a larger operation. While most forms of sex work are considered criminal in the US, a large part of the industry (including stripping, escort services, camming, and pornography) is regulated.

People who visit SWs come from all socioeconomic classes and are of all gender and sexual identities. They may be seeking intimacy, sexual satisfaction they can't find elsewhere, getting off without attachment or commitment, experimentation, lack of judgment, to fulfill a fantasy, to fill a void, to be accepted unconditionally, to dominate or be dominated, and many other things.

I know many straight men who visit or have visited SWs. Often they tell me that they struggle with finding their committed partners or wives sexually desirable, especially postchildbirth. This speaks to me about the need to dismantle and educate around the old "virgin and whore" myth and to connect intimacy with arousal. The trend has become especially prevalent as pornography increasingly influences our expectations for sexual experiences.

Alice Little is one of the top-earning legal sex workers in America, working out of the Moonlite Bunny Ranch in Nevada. She told me she works **"a lot with virgins that particularly want to have a good first experience, because they've seen all of these horrendous models that are put out there by Hollywood and TV, that aren't really representative of what consensual sex is. We aren't modeling healthy sex for people. Pornography isn't doing it. Hollywood isn't doing it. TV isn't doing it. How in the world are people supposed to learn this skill?"** This isn't without historical precedence. Around the world, many well-intentioned or monied fathers took their sons to visit SWs for their first time. In fact, it was not uncommon for Ivy League college boys back in the day to have a house account at the local brothel set up by a parent who didn't want a paramour to interfere with their son's studies or, worse, interrupt the inheritance plan.

I'm spelling out exactly what sex work means here because many conflate consensual sex work with sex trafficking. Trafficking largely means that someone has been transported to any labor sector through coercion, force, fraud, or violence. Trafficking, while it can be and is often experienced by SWs, occurs at much higher rates within agricultural and domestic labor than in the sex industry. Trafficking is illegal and immoral, and it should be prosecuted to the full extent of the law. Making sex work illegal overall does not stop sex trafficking; in fact, more often it increases the probability (more on this shortly).

The current state of sex work in America and most of the world is dismal. SWs face unsafe conditions, lack medical insurance or basic protections, and are largely scorned by society. I believe sex work should be legalized and regulated so that the health and safety of those who find themselves working in the sex industry can be maintained.

If you are wondering why or how someone might choose to work in such an unprotected labor force, let's consider some historical realities.

To start, up until the early twentieth century, most people born as women (and those who were born enslaved) had few occupational choices. Sometimes I muse about my fate had I been born in England in the Middle Ages; Italy during the Renaissance; or France during the Revolution. Likely, being a white woman born into an upper- or middle-class family and having a vulva would limit me to three options: become a housewife, devote my life to God, or become a sex worker.

Doubtless, I would not have the choice to marry for love but as a matter of class and circumstance. Then I would be someone else's property, and even if I was lucky enough to own a piece of land, it would automatically become my husband's. He could beat me or divorce me as he saw fit (or even label me a witch and have me burned at the stake). Even if I was an aristocrat's wife, there would be the chance of a beheading or a palace coup. In the best-case scenario, I might be locked up in a chastity belt while my husband went off to battle. If I was a nun, I would be confined in a convent, thus "protected" from male advances, and confined to spend my days among my own gender, with little or no interaction with secular society. As a sex worker, I'd face many challenges—from violence to mental and physical stress to basic disregard by other humans—yet I'd be able to have some degree of financial independence. Whatever role I was, my vulva would decide my fate.

In the twenty-first century, even with more professional options available to people with vulvas, SWs get into the industry for a host of reasons: to pay their bills, put food on the table, take care of their children, get housing, put themselves through college, caretake others, earn "easy" money (it's never easy), and many others. One friend told me that after leaving an abusive home life at fourteen, she was "turned out" by her girlfriend at the time, someone she loved, who introduced her to a way of supporting herself instead of being on the streets.

Sometimes poverty, abuse, or lack of education dictates sex work as the only opportunity that someone feels they have. When people are homeless or survivors of abuse, addiction, or domestic violence, sex work as an occupation is often referred to as "survival sex"— literally a way to participate in the street economy in order to make it another day.

I met my friend Catherine Clay at an event held by Dress for Success, a global nonprofit that empowers women with the tools to achieve economic independence. Now retired from the sex industry, Catherine told me, **"I come from a family that groomed the younger ones into this profession. As I look back, I know that there's just full support [for being a sex worker]. So that we've never been told, that's not something you shouldn't do. I've always been told that's what you should do and we should never be broke as long as we have that between our legs."**

In every other area of labor—especially in areas subject to trafficking, like immigration and domestic work—regulators consult with people who work in those sectors when developing safety measures and laws. However, SWs, voices are disregarded when it comes to regulations affecting their industry. In the United States this leads to the passage of bills that end up hurting the people they are supposedly designed to protect, like FOSTA-SESTA,[32] acronyms for

---

32 The intention behind these laws was to restrict and outright ban any and all websites and online content that facilitated sex trafficking. However, as a result of this policing, many sex workers and sex educators have been shadow banned on platforms like Instagram or completely kicked off of the Internet. Politically, *sex trafficking* and *prostitution* are synonymous terms, but in reality there is a large difference between sex trafficking (involuntary) and sex work (voluntary). These laws have put sex workers into dangerous positions, as they also have caused the shutdown of private digital networks they used to create and maintain a safe community; sex workers no longer have digital means by which to compare notes on prospective clients, share information on past (potentially violent) clients, or use private messaging features on social networks. With all of the virtual means of sex work taken away, sex workers must also go out into the world to advertise and gain new clientele. Without these resources available to them, meeting a prospective client in person, whom they have little to no references on, can cost a sex worker their life.

the Fight Online Sex Trafficking Act and the Stop Enabling Sex Traffickers Act, a package of federal laws that were passed in 2018.

I am going to get in the weeds here so I can walk you through how it is possible that something that was well-intentioned (stopping sex trafficking) can turn into something that does more harm than good *if* we don't include voices from within the marginalized communities affected, like SWs. FOSTA and SESTA are good examples of how technological advances and our collective desire to consume and participate in sexually explicit acts and content *without* open and inclusive dialogue has led to a massive mess and a lot of confusion about who the "good" and "bad" guys are.

In the past twenty years, just like most other industries, a lot of sex work has migrated online. The Internet has in many ways made it safer for SWs to prescreen and vet clients, create and share lists of "bad tricks," secure payment, and advertise off of the streets. It has also made it simpler for law enforcement to track illegal activity and potential sex trafficking.

As sex work has migrated online and pornography has exploded, we've seen the rise of more "acceptable" mainstream sites like OnlyFans, where you can pay for NSFW[33] photos and videos from a range of people—both people who consider themselves SWs and those who don't but who want to engage directly with fans. Rap superstar Cardi B has an account (as of this writing), and Beyoncé name-checked the site in a song with Megan Thee Stallion.

Obviously, no one (at least no one reading this book) condones child porn or sex trafficking. The problems with FOSTA and SESTA are that they don't appear to provide concrete avenues to purposefully stopping illegal sex trafficking, and they simultaneously make things murky in a number of areas. For one, they conflate consensual and nonconsensual sex work, which has had massive ramifications for those who use online platforms to work safely and/or present any kind of sexual material. While the bills ostensibly exist to stop people from advertising trafficked SWs on now closed-down sites like Backpage (immortalized in Janicza Bravo's 2020 film *Zola*), they also target websites like ours, The Sex Ed, that use the Internet to espouse sex education. On our Instagram account we even have to censor certain words in our posts, like *vagina* when we talk about periods or *orgasm* when we talk about sex-toy safety, because IG censors anything it perceives to be sex related as a result of these laws.

---

33 "Not safe for work."

While sites that openly contain sexually explicit material or talk about sex education are up for increased scrutiny, the bills don't hold mainstream sites accountable for sex trafficking, stalking, or revenge porn. According to a 2020 federal human trafficking report, more than half of online sex-trafficking recruitment that year took place via Facebook, which has zero verification processes in place for the accounts or media uploaded there. Instagram, which is owned by the same company, Meta (the rebranded name for Facebook as of 2021), has the same issue.

Anyone can easily post revenge porn or explicit content on mainstream social platforms with no consequences or laws to prevent them. Nor do the social platforms make it easy to report or get revenge porn taken down. Meanwhile, as attorney Carrie Goldberg points out,

> PornHub happens to be pretty aggressive when it comes to content removal. They're faster than Facebook or Twitter, the companies that we used to associate with upstanding companies doing the right thing. Companies that have the most resources often are the most slow to act. But PornHub has been super responsive, and they say, "Listen, we have enough porn. There's enough consensual porn. We don't need to be making money from nonconsensual porn. That's not good for the industry." They'll take stuff down without too many questions asked.

The above is something to think about when we read bills or opinion pieces from people who aren't inclusive of those who work within the sex industry and *want to be involved in creating change.* The state of affairs for sex work makes me think of another interesting double standard and area of hypocrisy. Cannabis is now decriminalized or legalized in almost all fifty US states. Like sex work, this is another industry with a high degree of incarceration for black and brown people. Yet with white investors and tech bros betting heavily on marijuana and lobbying for legalization, it is now commonplace to be able to buy cannabis over the counter in many states.

There's a hierarchy within the sex-work industry known as the "whorearchy." It is based on how close workers get to clients, how they conduct their business, and what kinds of stigma they face. This ideology, which assumes that some forms of sex work are "better" than others, has existed since the first known brothel temple in 2400 BC, which was run by Sumerian priests and dedicated to

Ishtar, goddess of love, fertility, and war. Workers in this brothel were classified in three categories. The highest grade were allowed to perform sex acts within the temple for those of high rank; the second class operated on the grounds and for visitors; and the lowest class found their customers on the streets.

Here's how the whorearchy breaks down today. Imagine a pyramid with cam girls, phone-sex operators, and anyone who doesn't perform sex acts face-to-face at the top. As we move down a level, there are strippers (though burlesque performers typically move up a level, as they have less audience interaction than they did in the early twentieth century). The middle level includes sugar babies, adult performers, and dominatrixes. The second to lowest level incorporates full-service sex workers who labor indoors or through a licensed establishment. At the lowest level are full-service sex workers who hustle on the streets. The late Mistress Velvet elucidated this point, telling me,

> I'm not a street-based worker, so I have the privilege of being able to
> have a website and post ads and do background checks on pay-for
> services for safety and then also maybe get my own hotel or rent
> from the dungeon, et cetera, et cetera. All of that comes into play
> with my pricing, and then because of that they also know that I'm
> in a certain price bracket of sex work. Versus if you're in the street,
> you don't have a website, you don't have a lot of access to safety, and
> you're engaging in sex work in the car, then it's a lot cheaper and it
> also could be a lot more unsafe.

Let's revisit the case of Hugh Grant, who was arrested for soliciting Divine Brown back in 1995. Grant paid a $1,180 fine, was placed on two years' probation, and had to complete an AIDS education class. He also had a momentary public embarrassment and minor career dent (from which he swiftly recovered). As for Brown? She also paid a fine of $1,150 (for parole violations), attended an AIDS education class, did five days of community service, *and* was sentenced to 180 days in jail. It is interesting that years later, barely anyone thinks "Hugh Grant" and remembers this story—he was allowed to move past the transgression (boys will be boys, right?) But once a sex worker, that stain remains forever.

Much of the historical slang for sex workers alludes to their being sullied or "broken" in some way: "tarnished angel," "soiled dove," "fallen woman," "woman of ill fame," "woman of ill repute." Trans activist and journalist Ashlee

Marie Preston said, "I had so much shame around being a sex worker, so much shame around everything that I had to do in the name of survival, losing my virginity as a sex worker, doing all of these things, that I didn't want to face it. I also didn't want anyone else, especially the cis-hetero community, judging me for decisions that I had to make."

I honestly don't remember a time when I didn't care about the lives and stories of SWs. Even as a kid I was fascinated by the subject. I always felt it was unfair that so many people throughout history (and today) would be doubly condemned by society even if they had little other choice but to go down this path. I used to wonder how and why I felt so impassioned to carry this torch for SW rights, and then I heard a story that solidified for me the realities of how children carry around their parent's baggage.

I'm going to tell you a story. One I hope you won't judge.

It was 2015, and my father had recently died. My siblings and I were in the process of putting the house he lived in, which my grandparents built in the early 1930s, up for sale. I grew up in the same bedroom my father had as a child. We were sorting through three generations' and over eighty years of memorabilia and memories over one long weekend. It was not fun. The days were endless as we cleared through boxes, closets, and drawers, deciding what keepsakes we wanted, what was getting donated, and what we would throw away. It was especially painful going through my dad's clothes. Just weird overall.

At the end of each day, we'd gather together for takeout, crack open a bottle of wine, and trade stories about our dad. As the liquor flowed, the stories tended toward the "what a lovable rascal" genre. I loved my dad deeply, but he was a complicated guy. Maybe one of the reasons I try to remain nonjudgmental when it comes to people's unique relationships to sex, love, and fidelity is that my father was a lover of women extraordinaire. From the time I was little, I was hyperaware of his extramarital affairs. It was kind of an open secret. I mean, I never discussed it with my mom, but my siblings and I did among ourselves. When I was young I was angry on her behalf, but as I got older I recognized that my father had a deep void when it came to love, which he conflated with sex. He wasn't the only man I knew who did so, either. Instead of telling their partner that they wanted to have other women (or men), men with these desires often shroud them in secrecy and shame, leading to lies and betrayals.

I loved my dad, so ultimately I accepted his need to cheat as something that was part of him. We all have our flaws; that's what makes us human. I knew who he was and that he loved me in all the ways he knew how. Anyway, returning to the weekend with my siblings, we were sitting around laughing about how much our father misbehaved, and someone said, "Remember how he got arrested for solicitation when you were an infant, Liz?" Everyone started laughing. Except me. I had never heard the story. No one ever told me. The only reason my older half siblings knew was that my dad was a public figure and the arrest was in the newspaper at the time (which is partially why I am sharing it here, not to smear his memory).

I didn't laugh, but I also wasn't surprised. In a way it made a lot of sense. Of course I would be compelled to write a book about nineteenth-century sex work in Los Angeles and found The Sex Ed. No wonder I would have a strong desire to champion SW rights. It literally was coded into my DNA. It didn't change how I felt about my dad, and I didn't judge him for it. Whether he did it regularly or just that one time, I have no idea. It really doesn't matter. I could see how it was just another method for him to find intimacy and comfort for the deficit he felt. I mean, the man was a lonely only child who had six kids! He did everything to create a big sense of love and stability around him, and it still wasn't enough.

Sometimes people need so much love and sex—more than their partner or family can give—that they have to pay for it. I was in a relationship with a man who told me very casually about visiting SWs with his buddies fairly regularly before we were together. I didn't judge that either, though I did ask questions about fair payment, and I had trouble when he denigrated women whom he paid for sex, as though that made them "less than." What all this illuminates for me is a need for us to have more of a cultural openness and—for straight men especially—to talk about this stuff aloud. To share the loneliness and the scarcity and the cavities we feel and be able to find acceptance. To express less disdain toward SWs. To find some way to honor the fact that when it comes to sex, things aren't always going to look like we might want them to. This means being conscious that the way we want to see the world (if that be love and light and sacred sex) doesn't necessarily reflect everything and everyone in it.

The more we ignore, denigrate, and sweep under the rug the uncomfortable and illegal parts of sex, the more opportunities we create for sex trafficking, for violence, for people to become statistics. I don't want to be unconscious of our collective shadow side; when we pretend things don't exist, then we cannot do anything to change them. If we can bring light into the dark areas, maybe we can envision a different system around sex work. I don't have the answers or the capability to provide systemic change here, just the desire to have more transparency and inclusive dialogue.

I want to leave you with some more words from Catherine Clay, who is one of the more empowered people I know:

> Having these conversations is what helped me feel I don't have to be ashamed to talk about prostitution. I have some friends at my mental health clinic job, and a lot of them have kids, but they're afraid to talk about sex. But when organizations are trying to give you housing, one of the only ways to get housing is if you talk about you being a prostitute. But it's taboo. No one wants to have this conversation. I'm a part of the Department of Mental Health. I'm the only former prostitute that gets to sit in on these meetings and advise them on how to outreach and engage with them. I also get to operate with the police department when they do prostitution stings. I get to talk to the prostitutes and offer them mental health [counseling]. It's an underground world that nobody really understands, unless you live in the world. It's a lifestyle that will eat you up and spit you out and [go on to] the next person, if you're not strong enough to survive. I just think having these conversations . . . is really important to bring awareness to it.

MENSTRUATION, MASTURBATION, AND MANIFESTATION

The more we can tap into the ancient wisdom of our bodies—including our fluids—and the more intention we practice in self-love (masturbation), the more we can channel our orgasms toward manifesting our deepest prayers and dreams.

In the previous chapters I covered foundational aspects of sexual health and how we can approach each of them mindfully. By now, I hope you have a greater sense of how your sexuality, or sexual energy, affects and is affected by every aspect of your existence.

The following chapters delve further into how we can integrate consciousness or spirituality within sexuality. I will be laying some esoteric ideas on you, but not everything can be explained by science. Aren't the great mysteries of the universe what keep us asking existential questions (and reading self-help and spirituality books)?

In the twentieth and twenty-first centuries, we have become out of tune and out of touch with our animal nature and intuition. We live in cities that are lit artificially, use digital alarms to wake us from slumber, clean ourselves from top to bottom with an arsenal of "hygienic" products, and for the most part actively avoid observing our bodily fluids.

Have you ever been to an acupuncturist, gynecologist, or a Western doctor? They may ask you about your bowel movements, menstrual cycle, and/or other bodily fluids in order to get a complete picture of your health. Not only do these fluids tell us about our physical health, they can also provide clues to our emotional and mental states.

Historically and culturally, in the Western world, menstruation has been viewed as a dreaded event rather than as a cause for celebration, exaltation, and reverence. For those of us who menstruate, during our cycle our bodies demand we pay attention, speaking loudly via often intense physical and emotional fluctuations. In the past, we may have labeled these shifts as bad or inconvenient. But what if we were to respect menstruation as a powerful time of creative flow and energy? A chance to turn inward and harness our extraordinary capacity for reflection, healing, intuition, and wisdom? Mirroring nature's rhythms and seasons of life and death, menstruation may not be the most comfortable experience, but it does heighten our sensitivity of mind, body and spirit.

Menstruation needs a massive PR overhaul.

Whether or not you bleed, getting familiar with menstruation is useful. Chances are, someone whom you love menstruates. Understanding more about what they go through each cycle will enlighten you and expand your empathy, too. A twenty-year-old heterosexual male friend of mine recently told me that he would *never* buy menstrual products for anyone (he has yet to fall in love). I bet him a thousand dollars that in the next ten years he would, either for his girlfriend, his sister, or some other pal. I also suggested that knowing more about the menstrual cycle would better inform him of what time of the month a partner is most likely to get pregnant and suggested that offering chocolate and menstrual-cramp-relief medication was a sexy move. He didn't take me up on the wager after our conversation.

If you menstruate, are you aware of the color, intensity, and consistency of your flow from month to month? If you use a menstrual cup, you may be more up close and personal with your blood than if using a tampon or pad. When changing or washing out your menstrual products, are you focused on cleaning up, or do you spend a little extra time examining your blood? Is it darker or lighter this month than last? Have you been going through any personal life stressors or changes? If you keep a journal, it could be interesting to note how your cycle shifts along with where you are at emotionally and spiritually.

Would you consider taking it a step further and dab a bit of your blood on your body in the shower? I'm not suggesting you go full *Midsommar* and run through a field naked and covered in menstrual blood (unless, of course, that is your fetish and you live out in the wilds where you can do so uninhibitedly and without freaking out your neighbors). But a little smear somewhere on your body for a few seconds before you wash it off is not going to hurt you. I know plenty of people who dump the contents of their menstrual cups in their garden to fertilize their plants, so a little smudge in the shower can give you just a taste of tapping into your animal nature.

Why even do all this, you ask? The more in touch we are with our body and blood flow, the more we can be empowered by our periods instead of dreading "that time" of the month.

Another thing to consider: Do you notice what phase the moon is in during your menstruation? Some bleed on the crescent moon, some on the full moon, some on the waning moon, and others on the new moon. The word *menstruation* comes from the Latin *mensis*, which means "month" and is also one of the roots for *moon*. The average menstrual-cycle length is around 29.5 days, and the lunar cycle lasts 29.5 days. It is okay if yours doesn't match exactly that cycle—with modern technology, birth control, hormones, and stressors, it is totally normal to be out of sync. To track your menstruation in relation to the moon cycle, simply begin to observe how it relates to the moon. Do you ovulate on the full moon and menstruate on the new moon? Or something different? Don't judge, just observe. Along with tracking what phase the moon is in, you might want to keep a journal of how you feel before and during your menstruation to get in the practice of noticing how your body tunes in with nature.

I've noticed that when I menstruate on the full moon—watch out! Everything becomes more intense, including my cramps. If I allow myself to tap into the feelings that arise, I feel more in sync with nature. One of my most powerful cycles happened while I was in Mérida, Mexico, during a full-moon solar eclipse on the winter equinox. I happened to have my period while visiting a sacred Mayan archaeological site, Dzibilchaltún. One of the structures there, known in English as the Temple of Seven Dolls, aligns perfectly with the sun during the equinox. Whether it was the moon or the power of the site or both, I have never bled so profusely nor with such debilitating cramps in my entire life. I recall lying on the floor back in our hotel room telling my partner, "I just want to lie on the ground and bleed into the earth, like the generations of women who bled before me." I was seriously out of my mind! But I also felt so alive, so potent and connected to the earth and my female ancestors. Thankfully he had enough emotional intelligence and appreciation of my eccentricities to humor my deeply felt experience. At that moment, even though the pain was overwhelming, I felt that I was part of something bigger and more mysterious than I could intellectually comprehend.

In many ancient cultures and mythologies, the sacredness or magic of menstruation was celebrated. Ancient Egyptians allegedly smeared menstrual blood on different body parts to act as a potent talisman to ward off evil or induce fertility; ancient Greeks mixed menstrual blood into the soil to help crops grow. Many cultures viewed (and still view) menstruation as a time that brings higher intuition, more vivid dreams, and greater spiritual insight. Lei Wann at the Limahuli Garden and Preserve told me it is believed, in Hawaiian cultural practice, that **"during menstruation you are receptive to the gods and elements. You are connected to the moon and tides and can go into their world. You flow with the tides and earth; you have the ultimate power of conceiving and birth. You are Hina, the moon goddess!"** Menstruation allows one to be more receptive to the mysteries and rhythms of nature. It can be a powerful time to go within, to meditate, to tune in to what your body is telling you.

What if we honored all the magical qualities of menstruation instead of concentrating on the ways it hinders us? We need to reframe the language we use around menstruation. I have been wanting to rebrand the phrase PMS forever! We will get to why in a moment. But first, let me break down the four main phases of the menstrual cycle with their correct names. *Menstruation* is the shedding of the uterine lining (i.e., what causes bleeding). Estrogen and progesterone levels are low. The *follicular stage* is the time between the first day of one's period and ovulation. Estrogen will rise as an egg prepares to be released. *Ovulation* happens around two weeks or so before menstruation starts and signifies the release of a mature egg from the surface of the ovary. When someone ovulates, they are more likely to get pregnant. The *luteal phase* occurs just after ovulation (when ovaries release an egg), right before a period starts. If the egg was fertilized during ovulation, that person's body will produce human chorionic gonadotropin (hCG) to thicken the uterine lining. If the egg is not fertilized, estrogen and progesterone levels will drop and prepare the uterus for bleeding.

The luteal phase is what has become known as PMS. This term, short for premenstrual syndrome, was first established in a 1953 *British Medical Journal* article by two doctors, Raymond Greene and Katharina Dalton. They defined PMS symptoms as including bloating, breast pain, migraine headaches, fatigue, anxiety, depression, and irritability. It wasn't until the 1980s, however, that PMS became part of popular lexicon, often used to describe a "hysterical" or "insane" woman acting irrationally. In fact, there were a couple of murder trials in Britain in the 1980s that reduced two women's sentences after they used their severe PMS as a defense!

Sometime between the 1980s and the early 2000s, "being on the rag," "riding the crimson tide," and "major PMS" were commonly used phrases. I have been on the receiving end of intended-to-be-insulting comments like "Are you on your period?" fairly frequently when moody or emotional. Or maybe you've heard someone say that people with periods can't make good leaders because they will spin out of control once a month? I wish that every human being could experience menstruation, even for two to six cycles, just to equalize and normalize the spectrum of physical and mental changes that those of us who bleed have to push through while going to work, exercising, running a business, performing brain surgery, arguing a legal case, or enacting any other daily routine.

When I found out that PMS wasn't even a commonly used phrase until the 1980s, I started thinking about what they called luteal-phase symptoms back in the day. This led me to wonder how much so-called female hysteria played into the marketing of PMS and the commercialization of related products to regulate it.

Hysteria is derived from the Greek *hystera*, or uterus. Prior to the twentieth century, physicians deemed "hysteria" the cause of a diverse range of symptoms for women, including fainting, nervousness, insomnia, irritability, loss of or excessive appetite and sex drive, and mood swings. This word was used to dismiss female suffering, independence, depression, and fatigue. According to the abstract for "Women and Hysteria in the History of Mental Health," a 2012 article in the journal *Clinical Practice and Epidemiology in Mental Health*, "Hysteria is undoubtedly the first mental disorder attributable to women, accurately described in the second millennium BC, and until Freud, considered an exclusively female disease. Over 4000 years of history, this disease was considered from two perspectives: scientific and demonological. It was cured with herbs, sex or sexual abstinence, punished and purified with fire for its association with sorcery and, finally, clinically studied as a disease and treated with innovative therapies."

"Hysteria" was such a common affliction up through the early twentieth century that a quick perusal of literature or the pages of old Sears catalogs will turn up countless heroines locked up with this mysterious illness and even more advertisements for products promising a cure. Surprisingly, hysteria was not linked to menstruation in cultural conversation (or lack thereof). Menstruation and sanitary care were not publicly discussed *at all* until well into the nineteenth century, and even then it was mostly via mail-order catalogs advertising sanitary belts, which were made of rubber to put around the hips and suspended by a belt between the legs.

It wasn't until the 1930s that scientists seriously began studying the menstrual cycle. In his 1931 scientific paper "The Hormonal Causes of

Premenstrual Tension," published in *Archives of Neurology and Psychiatry*, gynecologist Robert Frank made note of the association between negative mood and the menstrual cycle: "It is well known that normal women suffer varying degrees of discomfort preceding the onset of menstruation. . . . These minor disturbances include increased fatigability, irritability, lack of concentration and attacks of pain." Sounds a little like "hysteria," right?

Also in 1931, psychoanalyst Karen Horney described increased tension, irritability, depression, and anxiety in the week preceding menstruation in one of her patients, labeling her diagnosis as "premenstrual tension." Interestingly, Horney was a trained Freudian psychoanalyst but later rejected his psychosexual and penis-envy theories. Among the fourteen psychology papers she wrote between 1922 and 1937 are titles like "The Problem of the Monogamous Ideal." Talk about before her time!

If PMS has complex ties to a made-up disease ("hysteria") that was used to control and suppress women for centuries, isn't it time we reevaluate our dialogue around period literacy and monthly hormonal changes? My friend Erica Chidi refers to her premenstrual stage as her "luteal phase," which I believe takes the sting out. Funny how reclaiming and renaming things provides insight and empowerment.[34]

Whether using a period app or an old-school moon calendar to track your menstrual cycles, being conscious of what stage of your cycle you are in can create space to begin to *appreciate* your once-dreaded luteal phase. Maybe it's a time to carve out more reflective moments for yourself or to change up your diet or workout for a few days to better support your flow. Or even to make masturbation more of a daily practice: when you orgasm, your body releases dopamine and oxytocin, hormones that are natural pain relievers. Masturbation can also help draw blood to your pelvic area, which in turn will help improve your circulation. This can aid in easing menstrual cramps.

Just before and often during menstruation, sexuality and sensuality may be überheightened—*and not directed toward a patriarchal ideal of procreation*. If libido and sexual desire are indeed at a peak during this time of the cycle, orgasms may be intensified. Whether practicing solo or with a partner, sex has the capacity to take you to new heights of pleasure and experience.

---

34 One of the first commercially sponsored sex-ed short films was a 1946 collaboration between Walt Disney and the Kotex sanitary product brand entitled *The Story of Menstruation*. This cartoon, which was considered progressive for its time, detailed how to track a menstrual cycle and was apparently the first time the word *vagina* was heard in a film.

Period sex may not be everyone's cup of tea (it is *most definitely* mine) but it also can cause some messy accidents. Most of us don't have the foresight to plan ahead for period sex, using red sheets or confining it to the shower for easy cleanup. If you've ever found yourself scrubbing sheets in the middle of the night, I recommend a simple homemade cleaning solution provided to me by hockey-playing pals who've had years of experience cleaning up blood on the ice and on their jerseys. Just mix one-quarter cup of hydrogen peroxide with three-quarters cup of cold water. Pour this solution on the stain or soak the material in it before washing. Trust me, it works.

Personally I've found there's nothing that takes my cramps away like an amazing orgasm. I believe we should all be having more orgasms on a regular basis—with ourselves! I cannot promote masturbation enough, regardless of what kind of genitals you have and whether or not you menstruate. *Masturbation is literally self-love and the key to tapping into your sexual force.* If self-care equals self-love, then playing with ourselves is the ultimate act of combining both.

When we consciously value and eroticize our bodies and solo playtime, it serves on a superficial level to help us delve into a deeper meaning of gratification. Go ahead and caress those curves, stroke them balls, ritualize for yourself the experience you might fantasize a lover creating for you.

I would love for primary sex education to include teaching that it is healthy, natural, and normal to masturbate. Masturbation gives you autonomy over your own pleasure and body—before you put your fulfillment in other people's hands. Too many of us learned what got us off from someone else before we gave ourselves permission to explore our bodies. I have bought so many vibrators for adult female friends who tell me they don't have a masturbation practice. Sometimes they won't even open the box for months, but eventually I will get a call or text saying what a game changer it is. I recently had a conversation with a woman who told me that it made her uncomfortable hearing her teenage daughter say, "I'm so horny, I just want some dick" because she wasn't sure how to have a conversation around sex—and was worried about her daughter getting her heart broken by some fuckboy. I suggested she buy her a vibrator instead, thus empowering her to get off (and solving the horniness temporarily) without a partner. When we are dependent on someone else to make us cum, we often become less selective of our partners.

For males from their teens up through their late twenties or even early thirties, masturbating before dates or going out is not only healthy but also gives raging hormones a positive outlet. There are a number of popular masturbation device for penis owners, including the Fleshlight, which looks like a flashlight but has a flexible vaginal, anal, or mouth-shaped canal built in, made from proprietary mineral oil and rubber polymers to mimic human cavities. (Note: all sex toys should be cleaned properly after each use and not be shared except with your partners.)

It's funny, 'cause the things that can ground us and give comfort and bliss, like masturbation and meditation, which are *100 percent FREE and not dependent on anyone other than ourselves*, seem to be the most difficult for us to carve out time for.

Dr. Joycelyn Elders, who holds both an MD degree and a master's in biochemistry, became the first African American woman to hold the position of surgeon general of the United States in 1993. During her tenure, under then-President Bill Clinton, teenage pregnancy rates dropped, and accessibility to birth control, HIV tests, and breast cancer screenings was expanded. In the course of her time in office, Dr. Elders stirred up controversy with her strong stances in favor of comprehensive sex education, drug legalization, and increased abortion access. Only fourteen months into her tenure as surgeon general, Dr. Elders was forced to resign after suggesting that teens should learn to masturbate as part of safe-sex education during a speech she gave at the United Nations on World AIDS Day. Dr. Elders told me that

> my God and your God may be a different God, but my God feels
> that 99 percent of sex is for pleasure. I feel that God meant for sex to
> be wonderful, enjoyable, and pleasurable. I feel that God taught us
> how to masturbate. If he had never wanted us to touch ourselves or
> get any pleasure from masturbation, we would have never learned how.
> Parents should tell their children that there is nothing wrong with
> touching yourself. You aren't going to go crazy, you aren't going to go
> blind, you won't get a disease, and you know you're having sex with
> somebody you love. You're not going to get anybody pregnant. But the
> other thing, you should do it in the privacy of your own room. It's not
> to be done in public. It should always be done in private.

When and how did you first discover that touching your genitals gave you pleasure? Did your parents shame you for it or encourage you to explore your body? Did you talk openly with friends about masturbation styles? Do you currently maintain a regular masturbation practice, whether you are partnered or solo? I've found that many people will stop masturbating in a relationship or will feel uncomfortable if their partner self-pleasures. I do not understand this mindset at all. Do you stop exercising, working on your mental health, seeing your friends, meditating—whatever you do to maintain a sense of balance and calm—because you have a partner? Masturbation is no different.

Health benefits of masturbation include reduced stress, better sleep, improved self-esteem, and, often, the temporary release of muscle tension and menstrual cramps. During orgasm, endorphins, oxytocin, and dopamine are released, amplifying sensations of pleasure in your body and brain. As you reach orgasm, your body discharges DHEA, a hormone known to boost the immune system, improve cognition, and keep skin healthy. Penile orgasms release testosterone, which helps regulate sperm production, muscle strength, and sex drive. Furthermore, orgasms can also strengthen muscle tone in the genital and pelvic floor area, leading to better sex and stronger orgasms. All of this sounds great to me!

Mutual masturbation—either pleasuring oneself while in the presence of a partner who is simultaneously doing the same or both partners engaging in manual (often nonpenetrative) pleasuring of each other—is a great way to get to know a partner. It's much easier to please someone when they show you *exactly* how they like to pleasure themselves. Unfortunately, many of us still carry a lot of shame around masturbating, whether solo or in the presence of another person. Here are a couple of real-life examples of how that might manifest:

1. You are a healthy, sexually active man who loves to beat off to online porn, but when your partner asks you to show them how you masturbate, you freeze up. You feel uncomfortable and insecure. Perhaps your religious or cultural background has caused you to believe that touching yourself is an activity only done privately. Your partner is frustrated, and so are you.

2. You really want to orgasm, but your partner doesn't want to engage in sexual activity. You pull out your vibrator and get ready to go to town on yourself, but they look at you like you've got horns growing out of your head! You try to explain that you need to get yourself off and it has nothing to do with them, you're not asking for their help—but you feel guilty or ashamed of tending to your needs.

To me, these examples show how out of touch we tend to be with our animal nature. I swear my cat spends half the day licking his balls, and he seems pretty happy. So do babies who unselfconsciously tug on their penis or stick a finger in their vagina. Of course we become socially conditioned to understand these activities aren't for public view, but we also can't help absorb some of the self-conscious cues around playing with ourselves.

We also tend to put a lot of pressure on ourselves to climax when we masturbate. Masturbation can be considered self-care, like stretching, slowly putting on a moisturizer, or luxuriating in a bath. It's not about the end result but about the time we take to adore and fetishize ourselves.

To refute some common urban lore: you won't desensitize or overstimulate your genitals by regularly using your vibrator set on a single speed. (If you are seriously worried, you can try a new toy.) And *NO*, you won't grow hair on your palms if you masturbate too much. Antimasturbation myths such as these were widely propagated in the late 1800s by freaked-out physicians who claimed that most women were entirely frigid, with a tenth the sexual energy of men. Female orgasms (known then as "voluptuous spasms") were said to interfere with conception, and "impure thoughts" were to be suppressed at all costs. Doctors and reformers alike urged women to steer clear of romance novels, lest reading them caused blood to flow to the sexual organs and induced excessive excitement.

Such inane claims even made their way into the creation of the most American of products: breakfast cereal. Dr. John Harvey Kellogg, founder of the Kellogg's cereal brand, was a vehement antimasturbator. Kellogg created the original corn flakes recipe in 1878 as part of an overall diet plan for preventing sexual arousal by feeding children this "healthful" cereal each morning. He believed masturbation caused cancer of the womb, urinary diseases, nocturnal emissions, impotence, epilepsy, insanity, and mental and physical debility, among other ailments. Kellogg also advocated rehabilitation for masturbators, advising circumcision for boys and applying phenol, a carbolic acid, to young girls' clitorises. YIKES!

Masturbation should be touted with the same zeal with which people swear by exercise or meditation practices. I personally feel more empowered public speaking or negotiating business after I've attended to my own orgasm. It gives me an *edge*. If we can blend our meditation and masturbation practices, even better. I speak from experience that combining breath work, pelvic floor exercises, and masturbation can lead to transcendent bliss.

In order to achieve this, it is important to start a masturbation practice. I am specifically calling it a "practice" because we want to be *intentional* with the time and not just bust a quick nut. Every once in a while, can you make masturbation (your self-love time) a ritual?

If the mere thought of masturbating makes you uncomfortable, you can start simply. For example, begin with a body scan. Lie down in a comfortable position and start to notice how your body feels. Breathe into your feet and toes, working your way up to your knees, inner thighs, pelvis . . . you can even skip your genitals and move up to your belly button, nipples, and clavicles . . . eroticize yourself. If you find yourself drawn to a particular body part, spend more time breathing there, and you can touch, stroke, or massage yourself there, too. The point is to put into practice getting to know how incredibly amazing and powerful your body and sexual energy are.

Another option is to put on or take off whatever makes you feel most erotic, horny, sensual, or primal. Set the mood as if you are seducing a lover. Maybe that means lighting a candle and putting on a playlist that you've created with a specific mood in mind. If music isn't your thing, it could be pregaming with a sweaty workout, a long bath, a delicious meal, a glass of wine, or a joint—really anything that gets your endorphins flowing and makes you *slow down* to connect to your body.

As you masturbate, imagine yourself receiving all the sex energy you may normally reserve for a partner. If you want better sex with another person, it all starts with loving up on yourself! If you'd like to do a masturbation ritual together with your partner, take turns creating an erotic atmosphere and observing as you show each other how you would get off if you were alone. Not only will it be spicy, it'll likely be educational for you both as well.

So now, how do we tie all of the above together to *manifest through orgasm*? This might sound a little freaky, but it is really very simple: the energy of your own orgasm plus intention *equals power*. We are clear at this point that sexual energy is potent, which is why we want to develop more consciousness around how we understand and direct it, right? So imagine that your orgasm is one of the *most powerful expressions* of this energy. It's like focusing all your attention on your five-thousand-horsepower engine to leave all the other cars in the dust. So if we are connected to our bodies, if we are aligned in mind, body, and spirit, we can channel this might to higher purposes and use our orgasms for empowerment.

There's a French expression for an orgasm, *la petite mort*, which translates as "the little death." This refers to the post-orgasm stage, when your consciousness is weakened and which may even feel like a spiritual release. Have you ever felt out of your body after a strong climax? If you meditate or pray, maybe you have experienced a different kind of transcendence after an orgasm when for even a moment you feel divinely connected. That moment of orgasm or transcendence looks and feels different for each of us, just as colors and textures do.

It might seem silly to wish upon a star or light a candle in a place of worship or on a home altar—or these may already be part of your usual routine. Perhaps you have a certain ritual when your favorite sports team is playing or a visualization technique you use when you are interviewing for a new job. Manifesting through orgasm is not all that different. You can even incorporate aspects of the spiritual traditions you already maintain. It just means bringing mindful awareness of what you are looking to manifest into a sensual realm. Remember the training montages set to stirring music in the *Rocky* movies, where the hero directs all his focus toward becoming the best fighter? Using your orgasm to manifest is kind of like that, but the goal can be specific ("I want to make more money, buy a house, get a better job, love my body more") or mystical ("I want to connect to the universe, feel deeply at peace, be at one with nature").

The more affirmations of positive self-acceptance and self-love you can include as you manifest—that is, masturbate—your way to orgasmic release, the better! Visualize in your mind or repeat aloud what it is that you are desiring as you self-pleasure. Don't trip out if you don't orgasm (remember, it's not always the goal). Just the act of putting all this attention toward manifesting through sexual release is 80 percent of the work.

Ashley Manta, a pleasure and intimacy coach, calls manifesting through orgasm "sex magic." She defines it as "pleasure-fueled alchemy" and says that **"through solo practice, sex magic has allowed me to fast-track my personal growth and professional success. I have become my favorite lover, something I never thought I'd be able to say. I've learned how to use my energy to access extraordinary pleasure. I've shed my shame about my fantasies, and I've come into a deeply loving relationship with my body."**

The ecstatic release of neurotransmitters and hormones during orgasm or heightened sensual play can be sacred or even supernatural. Honestly, it's like trying to describe what a rainbow feels like. This all may sound a little hippie-dippie acid-trippy, but there wouldn't be legends of ancient and religious texts devoted to the transcendent power of orgasm if there wasn't something here. How you manifest it personally is up to you. All it takes is being open to exploration.

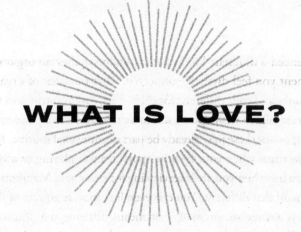

WHAT IS LOVE?

What is *love*?
How do we give *love*?
How do we receive *love*?
What do we expect from *love*?
What exactly is self-*love*?
How can we cultivate more *love*?

Although I've experienced many different kinds of love over my life thus far, in the past few years, my definition of *love* has been entirely upended. I used to think love was something that existed outside of me, that in order to experience love, one needed to be validated and loved back by another person or people.

If I'm honest, as much as I preached the practice of self-love to others personally and professionally, I didn't realize how much work it would take to truly love myself. Nor did I know how to surrender *fully* to love. I didn't truly show up for love or give it without expectation and conditions. I have since come to realize that love for self, community, nature, and the greater good is essential to our understanding of the depths of what love can be.

Our shared definition of love tends to be wrapped up in romantic and sexual ideals. Most of us associate love with romance, sex, partnership. We may be accustomed to love affecting or afflicting us by causing us to obsess on our object of affection or to desire to possess and claim someone as our own. We might willingly and wholeheartedly declare ourselves to another or reject them fully if love is unrequited or hurtful. Popularly speaking, the idea of love makes us think of riding intoxicating highs and the opposite of that, experiencing debilitating lows. Most love songs, books, poetry, and art about love celebrate these extreme states.

Dr. Walter Brackelmanns used to tell me that **"being in love is a transient psychotic state you have to get over in order to have a real love relationship with another person."** Love can make us feel completely bonkers, as our body and brain react to the chemical rush of being attracted to someone. Research on the first stages of love and cocaine addiction shows that both cause increased activity in the brain and nervous system, as well as intensified nervous system arousal as dopamine and norepinephrine surge. They also both link pleasure to desire (for sex or coke), sleeplessness, euphoria, and loss of appetite. Cocaine addiction and falling in love can induce obsessive behavior. New lovers tend to think about each other 95 percent of the time, as would someone jonesing for their next fix. Love can feel like an addiction—hence the expression "Love is a drug." Withdrawal symptoms in our brains from both cocaine and opioids can also mirror the effects of heartbreak from romantic love.

When I think back to my first love, at thirteen years old, I associate the feeling with losing myself: failing all of my classes that semester; talking on the phone with him every night until the sun came up; being sleepless, disoriented, and crushing on him beyond measure. I changed my schedule, priorities, and desires to suit the romance. I was utterly intoxicated, bewildered by his eyes and locks of hair falling over thick brows. He was the first superdreamy Peter Pan bad boy I lost my heart to (unfortunately, not the last). I thought I would die without him. It may have been my teen hormones going wild, but I was madly, crazily in love. I discovered perception-altering drugs (LSD and cannabis) around the same time as I was exploring this new feeling. Both my infatuation and the highs were blissful escapism; I felt like I was transcending, surrendering to alternate universes. Reflecting on it now, I see how linked the feeling between love and drugs was for me, the feeling of being engulfed in a temporary state followed by some kind of crash. Now love feels more like sinking into a warm bath in a lover's embrace than completely forgetting myself.

Maybe you can relate to this? Or have a friend or family member who becomes so wrapped up in a new love that they change their habits, check out from other activities and relationships to the point that they become someone else? This is typical of the accepted love feeling that we tend to celebrate in popular culture and come to *expect* when we meet a potential partner. That immediate *holy fuck I'm so overwhelmed I can't see straight my knees are buckling and stomach's in knots I can't be without them* predicament.

The state of being in love, or limerence, lasts roughly two to four years. As oxytocin floods your brain, it is a feeling of being high and marked by infatuation and anxiety. Over time, a romantic relationship changes as lust decreases. Hopefully, bonding and, in Walter's terms, a "dialogue of intimacy" take place—a communication of feelings and insecurities. Romantic love sustains a relationship over time. As does regular sex, an important part of intimacy. This is not the Disney version of love where Cinderella (or insert any princess myth here) and Prince Charming ride off into the sunset and live happily ever after. As Walter put it, **"If you want to be 'in love' for the rest of your life, you have to keep rotating partners every one to four years."** Real love begins when they shack up in the castle and have to deal with their respective idiosyncrasies, evolution, and extended families. All of which takes enormous determination and consideration on the part of both parties.

Growing up, the idea of love for many of us was wrapped up in a mentality of being saved, fixed, rescued, or healed by a romantic partner. The cultural viewpoints and media I absorbed presented a "perfect love" to aspire to—"Someday your prince will come" and all that nonsense that many little girls were raised on. It's almost as though we learn to fall in love with an image, with the potential of who someone could be, rather than who they really are. Man, did it take me years to undo that programming. I used to think love meant presenting the best possible version of yourself, not letting that mask slip or allowing yourself to be *seen*.

For the first season of The Sex Ed podcast, I asked fifty strangers what they thought love was. Their definitions, while wildly diverse, all focused on romantic and sexual love:

- "I've said it to six people, and I meant it every time."

- "I've been married twice; it's my second marriage. I'm very much in love with my husband. I [also] have a girlfriend that lives a couple hours north, and I love her a lot. I just haven't been able to tell her the words, but I think about it all the time."

- "I've definitely been in love with, like, idealized mental models of people. I'm trying to fall in love with actual real people."

- "It's harder when it comes to queer, male-bodied people finding that kind of intimacy. I mean, obviously sex is easy to come by. But finding softness isn't something that's openly encouraged. So it's more a question of whether there were times I have found intimacy, whether it's shared mutually or if it's something like a romanticization or a crush. So it's always unclear in that regard. Could I ask you, how you know if someone loves you back?"

- "I think a younger me back in my twenties thought that love was about sex. And then as you get older and become wiser, you realize that it has nothing to do, in my opinion, with sex. It has more to do with giving and taking and being good and kind and [having] respect. Love is definitely respect."

- "It's the only thing that matters. And I don't have enough of it. I have a wife, we're not always in love. But I definitely felt a profound experience when I met her and we fell in love. And I still feel that little kernel of that is still there with her. It's not totally gone, thank God, but it definitely dims. And then it explodes. And then it's down."

- "I don't want to die alone. I have this fear of just being this cat lady and then dying. And then no one finds my body for two weeks. And then, like, my cat's eaten my nose and ears. If there is such a thing as 'the one,' to connect with that person, that's the challenge then, right? So the one is out there. There's someone for everybody. How are you supposed to find that person? Do you find 'em on fucking Tinder? That's what I'm doing. It's not working. But I'm trying. Even though I have no hope, I still try."

For something so central to human existence, it seems like none of us have much clarity around what love is. Most self-help books, Internet therapists, and Instagram experts devoted to love focus on helping people find someone to partner, have sex, and potentially procreate with. They may talk about love languages or how to care for and receive affection, but rarely do they define love. It's more a game-of-love mentality (how to possess, win, achieve) than an exploration of how to pursue a deeper understanding of love that links mind, body, and soul. So many people (I hear this particularly from men) would rather run from intimacy and love than face the possibility of feeling hurt, experiencing rejection, and revealing their deeper selves.

Still, the longing for love remains.

As much as we want love, we also live in fear of it: love is a risk and carries the possibility of pain. We may also fear that someone won't love us for who we really are. If we don't love ourselves first, we may maintain emotional distance from lovers as a defense mechanism, even in long-term committed relationships.

How did you first learn to love? Who taught you how to love yourself? Anyone? Were there adults around who loved themselves? Most often, our attraction to others is based on our wounded child self, reflecting the traits we have disowned and need to accept in ourselves. We may use someone else's love to heal our wounds or to fill our void. We may even jump from relationship to relationship without ever loving ourselves. We come to seek out "love" relationships that mirror our early childhood conditioning—until and unless we can break free from the patterns that keep us stuck repeating unhealthy ideals of love.

How we give and receive love as adults is informed by our primary caregivers and their character tendencies. The very ways in which your primary caregiver may have felt lacking in love or particularly judgmental about themselves would likely have been projected onto you as their child. So, for example, if your parent was unhappy about their body, they might have fixated on yours; or if they had insecurity around intelligence, they may have been overly worried about your grades. If you were abandoned or rejected by a caregiver, you may end up seeking emotionally unavailable partners. If your caretaker was overly enmeshed and smothering, it may cause you to feel distant and uncomfortable with overt displays of affection or intimacy.

Maybe you experienced a primary caregiver's love that was connected to shame or criticism in the name of "helping" or "disciplining" you. Maybe their love was neglectful, hurtful, or abusive. Perhaps their affection was overwhelming to the point that you felt suffocated by their love. It could be that you learned there were conditions and expectations around love—if you got good grades, behaved well, achieved this or that, or performed as expected, then you would receive love. It might be that your caregiver's attitude toward you swung wildly from cold and emotionally unavailable to possessive and effusive. All of these experiences teach us what we think is love and how to respond to it.

It's good to remind ourselves that the way we learned about love comes from the way our caregivers learned how to love, too! Remember the trauma chapter and how far back all of this goes? Although it's demanding, we have to do the work of individuating ourselves from our caregivers—and of loving others (including one's own children) with enough freedom to allow them to develop without living up to or fixing our baggage.

No one ever said love was easy.

We ought to be teaching the art of falling in love with ourselves before we give love away. So many of us learn the false belief that another's love and approval will make us whole or healed. That our pain, anger, sadness, or loneliness will be solved by the right person or outside circumstance. When the truth is, if we don't actually love ourselves, how will we have enough love to share? How will we be able to discern what type of love or relationship situation is best for us if we just accept whatever comes along because it's better than nothing, better than being alone?

Imagine being so blinded by love for yourself that you find even your weaknesses beautiful. Dazzled by your body's miraculousness, grateful every day for all the ways in which you are unique. Loving all your vulnerabilities as you might love those parts of another. What if we saw ourselves as a beautifully decorated, icing-laden cake, with romantic love simply the cherry on the top? Can you talk to your body about all the things you love about it? If you've never spent time looking at your genitals in a handheld mirror, consider this your prompt to do so. You can also stand in front of a bigger mirror, naked, and check yourself out. Sound cringey? Why? Because you wish you had smaller thighs, a larger penis, less cellulite? Can you even love up on the dimples on the back of your thighs or your cute little muffin top? Our bodies are miracles, but we often talk about the things we hate or want to change about them instead of what we love. It may be hard to do this exercise, but being able to see past the conditioning of the stories we've told ourselves about our bodies is where self-love begins.

I grew up in Hollywood, literally the epicenter of media mythology, which totally distorted my view of love, especially *self-love*. I come from a show-business family. My paternal grandfather produced one of the first feature films in Hollywood back in 1914 and went on to found multiple movie studios. My paternal grandmother was an actress and sometime *Vogue* model. All of my immediate and most of my extended family, in one capacity or another, are in the biz. My childhood was very privileged and definitely not normal by any standard. The majority of the people I grew up with or their relatives were actors, directors, producers, musicians, or otherwise associated with the industry. It was a highly concentrated petri dish of "special" people. I use "special" here not because I believe some people are more significant than others, as we are all unique, but because the outside world tends to place a high value on those who are in the public eye, which confers a very weird sense of "specialness" upon certain people. It all creates a warped sense of reality.

Because of this childhood perspective, I had a bird's-eye view of love as wrapped up in narcissism and celebrity—where culture seems to be now. We reward money, fame, and power with love. My dad used to say, "You're only as good as your last picture," and dinner-table talk often involved which movie or person had the highest box office numbers that week. By this standard, how "good" you are is measured by outward success. The unconscious lesson I learned growing up this way was that validation and worth came through placing ourselves and others on a pedestal. Everything revolved around being in the center of the spotlight or worshiping those who were. If we revere seeing ourselves reflected through the admiring gazes of others, we essentially allow others to dictate whether or not we are lovable.

From a very early age I witnessed adults around me caught in an intricate web of toxicity around love. To the outside world, the Academy Awards hoopla is one of the most glamorous things about Hollywood. You know what I would see and feel during that time of year? The Hollywood hierarchy on display in full force—you can literally smell the dysfunction, insecurity, and hustle. It was people looking around the room and not in your eye when they were talking to you, trying to see who else was there, who was more important, who might help further their career. I have had people I knew very well completely ignore me until they saw me speaking with someone famous and then make a beeline in my direction. Or the opposite: clearly killing time with me while glancing over my shoulder, abruptly breaking off in the middle of a sentence and leaving when someone more fabulous appeared. It felt fucking shitty. My self-esteem and worthiness would plummet, and I'd immediately start comparing and despairing about all the ways I didn't measure up. Even the most well-adjusted person in the world would have trouble maintaining self-assuredness within this microscopic lens of superstardom.

As proud as I am of my lineage, I am also deeply conflicted about being part of a legacy that has contributed to placing fame and fortune above compassion, community, honesty, and humility. I'm not saying I didn't have any positive modeling around love as a kid or that most of the people I grew up with had unhealthy values—in fact, my dad worked really hard to keep us grounded within the glitz that surrounded my upbringing. There are also many down-to-earth, "regular" folks in the industry (or as regular as one can be in such an environment). But honestly, being surrounded by all this "me, me, me" and "fame fixes everything" thinking impacted my sense of self-love.

Unfortunately, this has become the norm to emulate. With the domination of Instagram, reality TV, and social media influencers, many millennials, Gen Zers, and younger kids are growing up in an even more commodified culture saturated with higher-than-ever levels of narcissism and with the notion of love tied to external validation. Today our worth is measured by "likes" and comments, engagement across platforms. It's fucking exhausting. Sometimes I drive around Los Angeles and look at all the billboards advertising this or that product with perfectly-preserved-at-twenty-one skin and supertight bodies, and for a moment I lose faith in humanity. Celebrity has become the goal, but beyond financial gain is the very real desire for love. Public acclaim and acceptance more and more are supposed to fill the void of a lack of self-love. Where does this leave us? How does it help us evolve our love and acceptance of ourselves and others?

Which brings us back to the question: What is love, anyway? Great philosophers, poets, musicians, and authors have been striving to answer this for centuries. The person I think has come closest to encapsulating the modern complexities and mysteries of this elusive term is the late, great bell hooks, in her treatise *All About Love*, which I cannot recommend enough. I reread it every so often to remind myself that many other people out there are striving to redefine how we approach love. Yet the term itself, *love*, remains impossible to condense in a sound bite as our experience of it changes from year to year, relationship to relationship, the more we get to know ourselves and expand our capacity for love.

I never was as touched by the profoundness of love songs until I was going through my divorce, spilling tears while listening to Neil Young's *On the Beach* and the Zombies *Begin Here* on repeat. I realized then how much of the music I cherished was centered not around the exaltation of great love but around heartbreak. Have you ever loved someone so much that losing them through breakup or death hurt beyond a pain you could imagine? Have you ever been so wounded by love that you didn't think you would ever love again? We develop a muscle memory around love, scars that crisscross our heart, which can hold us back from believing in its power.

A few years later, I was in a blissed-out love bubble playing Al Green albums over and over. I listened to his early romantic love songs from the perspective of his later love of God. This led me on another spiral of thinking about love and the way it makes us feel. Was his love for God greater than that for his previous lovers? Were they one and the same? Was there a spiritual ideal of love to strive for? Is true love achievable only if the secular and sacred are aligned?

Thinking about love through an integrated perspective of sex, health, and consciousness (or mind, body, and soul) led me to face the reality that I needed to get my libido under control. It had always led to my decision-making about entering relationships, to my "falling in love." I wanted to move beyond the surface level of manifesting love as physical and sexual desire and instead to create the possibility of deeper spiritual bonds with myself and others.

Love is so much more than great sex and shared interests. Love is freedom and spiritual growth; it is expansive, evolving, and plentiful.

Love is radical honesty with ourselves and those we love. We are mostly wired to want to receive love, but love is giving freely without expecting it in return. Love is gestures of unconditional nurturing, kindness, and compassion. Love is generosity toward others, toward community, toward the planet at large. Love is inclusive. If you suffer, I suffer. Love is service.

Love is facing your shadows and embracing them. Love is accepting others for who they are—shadows and light, all of it—and not trying to change them. Remember the void we talked about earlier? We have to love it in others the way we must love it in ourselves. This was a hard one for me. I had to let go of falling in romantic love with what I saw as someone's potential and a false presumption that my love could make them change into a version of themselves better suited to what I desired in a partner. I see now that my failure to love people exactly as they showed up stopped me from *seeing and being seen* in love. Ego is a bitch, right?

Love is patience and constant effort. We can't cruise-control love. Love is work. And it's difficult work at that! It's so much easier to coast on good sex and nice companionship than to dig deeper into love.

There's a freedom and expansiveness to loving. When we love someone, we want to nourish their expansion as a human being. Love is making sacrifices (we can rephrase these as "offerings") without scorekeeping. Love is expressing gratitude for someone's mere existence. Love is encouragement. Love is putting ourselves out there with no guarantees.

Love is practicing differentiation, dancing the dance between togetherness and autonomy, as we grow together and as individuals. Love is without attachment to what things "should" look like or have looked like; love leaves room for the people we care for to become the best version of themselves.

I spent most of the year while writing this book living in Hawaii, where I witnessed radical acts of love on a daily basis. In a language that has hundreds of words to describe different winds,[35] the word for "love," *aloha*, is not only used to say hello and goodbye but has a much deeper meaning.

With the help of Hawaiian friends, I came to understand aloha as being present to an exchange of generous, loving energy. Broken down by each letter:

A stands for *ala*, or "watchful alertness."
L stands for *lokahi*, which means "harmonize" or "working with unity."
O stands for *oia'i'o*, meaning "truthful honesty."
H stands for *ha'aha'a*, or "humility."
A stands for *ahonui*, or "patient perseverance."

I came to see aloha as expressing the truth of one's spirit, being gentle with ourselves and others, a detached, nurturing, unselfish love—one that is calm, accepting, warm, strong, and tender. It made me think about how to be more consciously and outwardly loving, without reservation or fear—and to expand that love to strangers, to nature, to humanity. To perform more acts of unconditional love.

To practice aloha, we have to be able to ground ourselves first in a place of self-love. Much like on an airplane, where they announce that you have to put the oxygen mask on yourself before helping others, the same applies for love: loving your body, loving your void, loving and honoring your inner wisdom.

All of this reflecting on love and its transformative power pushed me to tap more deeply into my intuition. Before we get further into how honing our intuition is so valuable to every aspect of our lives, let me clarify that this is not a New Age concept! Great minds and logical thinkers have stated the importance of honoring our intuition for centuries. In his book *Pensées,* the seventeenth-century French physicist, philosopher, and mathematician Blaise Pascal wrote, "The heart has its reasons, which reason does not know. . . . We know truth, not only by the reason, but also by the heart."

Within our hearts lies an inner oracle. Often it just "knows" things our brains cannot rationalize. This "knowing" lies between our conscious thoughts

---

35 The mischievous wind that stole one of the composition notebooks I wrote this chapter in and threw it in a stream is known as *makani kolohe.* The least threatening (but distracting) wind I observed is called *nakeke*, or "wind that rattles with no purpose." I hear it as the distinct chatter of small talk at a cocktail party.

and our unconscious mind. Sometimes we also feel or "hear" these messages in our gut. When something is off but we can't place our finger on what exactly, it may be expressed as a sharp pang, a tightening or loosening of the bowels, an uncomfortable sinking feeling— like the expression "My stomach dropped." We all have the innate ability for somatic awareness inside, but it is usually drowned out by mental noise and societal conditioning. Or by what other people think is "best" for us and how we are expected to behave.

Gavin de Becker is considered one of the world's leading security specialists, primarily for governments, large corporations, and public figures. Intuition and how essential it is to our survival is at the center of his first book, *The Gift of Fear: Survival Signals That Protect Us from Violence.* As de Becker writes, "Intuition is always right in at least two important ways: It is always in response to something. It always has your best interest at heart."

In this book, de Becker highlights the importance of intuition after a lifetime of witnessing and working with victims and survivors of traumatic events, generally involving extreme violence or sexual assault. Many of the stories he recounts include examples of ways that we are programmed to ignore our inner guidance, either because it seems "illogical" or in order to be "polite" (often the case with women.) "Every day," he says, "people engaged in the clever defiance of their own intuition become, in mid-thought, victims of violence and accidents. So when we wonder why we are victims so often, the answer is clear: It is because we are so good at it."

While writing this chapter I had a conversation with a friend who had recently been assaulted by a naked man in a gender-specific public restroom (she was unharmed, thank goodness). She told me that she felt something was off when she entered the restroom: there were COVID policy signs on the stalls asking people to use every other toilet, but someone was in the one next to hers. She also noticed they had their pants pulled all the way down to the floor, which struck her as odd. But, like so many of us, she ignored these warning signals her intuition was sending.

Even after reading de Becker's book, my logical, rational mind continued to dismiss red flags arising from my gut and heart. That is, until I had an accident that landed me in the hospital— all because I ignored my intuition. I mentioned this incident previously in the chapter "Trauma," calling it a "freak accident in my garden."

I love plants. When my father passed away in 2015, I transplanted twenty-six rosebushes from his house into temporary pots and spent the better part of a year looking for a home for my roses while they lived at a friend's house. It was the roses that guided my home purchase. In 2017, I moved into my first-ever house of my own, having always lived in apartment buildings. I spent a good deal of time working on making my dream garden just so.

As I worked with a landscaper to complete the final stages of the garden, close friends gave me the housewarming gift of a lemon verbena tree. The tree was heavy, and it took two of us to put it in the back of my car so I could drive from their house to mine. My landscaper happened to be at the house when I arrived and took it out of the car for me while I climbed the forty-plus stairs from the street to my front door with other bags. Maybe thirty minutes later I came back outside to see that he had already planted the tree.

I felt sick to my stomach when I saw where it was: down a narrow sloping hill at the base of the fence to the street, with a water pipe running along the edge of the path and the eave of the garage three feet overhead.

Never before in my life had I experienced such a strong reaction to where something was planted. It just felt really off. Perhaps six times I said to him, "The tree doesn't want to be planted there. It feels precarious. It doesn't want to be there." But he was an older man who knew more about gardening than I did and insisted it was a good spot. So I dismissed my intuition, which had mostly served me well.

Ten days later, on the eve of a business trip to New York, with multiple people in my house, I decided to go cut some lemon verbena leaves from my tree to make tea for everyone.

Getting down to the tree was as tricky and precarious as I had imagined. I thought to myself, *Why on earth would he think to plant this here?* I had to reach up on my tiptoes to cut the leaves with the scissors. As I was coming back down to my heels, I slipped on the dirt and fell backward. I saw my bones pop out from my shin, and that is when I stopped looking down.

Why did I listen to someone else when I had such a powerful internal warning signal? Why couldn't I believe in myself? As de Becker writes, "Even when intuition speaks in the clearest terms, even when the message gets through, we may still seek an outside opinion before we'll listen to ourselves." It can be challenging to trust ourselves enough not to let others pressure us into doing things that don't instinctually feel right. Other people may have the best intentions when they give advice, as was the case with my landscaper, yet we really do know what is right for us. We are just excellent at second-guessing our inner wisdom.

Much of our self-doubt comes from a lack of self-love and self-esteem. The practice of self-love involves much more than eating well or meditating or writing in a journal. We have to dig deep into our uncertainty and learn to love and trust ourselves. Even and especially so when our intuitive guidance flies in the face of conventional wisdom and what everyone else is doing.

There is truth to be gained by listening to our heart and gut centers. I get calls all the time from friends asking me to help them make decisions. (They tell me it is "because you are so intuitive.") In each and every case, when I am asked for advice, the person asking already knows what is best for them—they just need to be reminded to tap into their instinct. I am not a psychic. I have learned by trial and error to tune in, and you can, too.

Here's a simple, grounding heart exercise to try the next time you are trying to figure out the correct way to move forward regarding a situation, person, or question. Settle comfortably into a quiet place and close your eyes. Take a few full body breaths—however many you need until your breathing changes from shallow to deep. Now ask your question aloud or silently and listen carefully to your body's response. Does your breathing or pulse change? Is it quicker, more frantic? Do you feel on edge or jittery? Do you feel like you have a stomachache or have to use the bathroom? Is your chest tight? Is there a slight constriction in your lungs or breath? Do you feel sadness, fear, guilt, or anxiety? Any of these signals from your body could indicate a red light—a no.

Or are your pulse and breath steady? Do you feel warmth or a sense of calm in your chest and stomach? When you ask yourself this question or think of the person or situation, do the corners of your mouth move up into a smile? Does your body feel relaxed? What is your heart telling you? The more we train ourselves to notice how we *feel*, the better we can react *in the moment*—whether in business or leading up to a sexual situation or in the bedroom—by attuning to the truth of our heart logic.

In a romantic relationship, this practice can be especially helpful. When we argue or face uncomfortable situations with a partner, we might tend to go easily into shutdown or resentment. Can we learn to pause and notice our ego overriding our heart? Can we reconnect with our heart center before engaging? As the author Madeleine L'Engle once said, "Your intuition and your intellect should be working together . . . making love. That's how it works best."

Imagine if individually and collectively we listened to our intuition and acted from a place of *love*. Once I located consciousness (or intelligence) in my heart, the more confidence I had in making major decisions based on what *felt right* versus what my head told me was logical.

The more that I lead from my heart, the more love I feel and receive in all aspects of my life. I try to practice more loving-kindness these days toward myself and others—especially when I am feeling irritated or triggered. It's definitely a meditation, not always a comfortable one.

Love is challenging, even if you are with or meet a "soul mate."

Are soul mates even real? Is it like searching for a unicorn? I once asked Walter Brackelmanns if he believed in soul mates. He told me he did, though he stressed how very rare it is to find someone with whom your psychopathology fits perfectly. Among his patients, he counted one case. Keep in mind he had been teaching for fifty years and had ninety-seven thousand hours of clinical practice under his belt. In Walter's view, you can have problems in your partnership and still be soul mates. A couple came in to see him because the husband was "fucking sex workers. . . . It got out of hand, so he told her what he was doing. And she got really upset." Walter excused the wife from therapy—the husband had individual issues unrelated to the marriage that needed to be addressed. Although it sounds baffling that Walter termed this couple to be soul mates, one can never judge the specifics of someone else's relationship, and it is indeed possible to have sexual needs outside of your primary partnership and still on every other level be spiritually and emotionally compatible.

We all know the common myths about soul mates: that we will meet and it's perfect love at first sight; the road will be smooth and paved with roses; the love will last forever. The reality is, finding someone with whom we can experience unconditional love, mutual respect, understanding, and a deep connection of mind, body, and spirit is no easy task. If we aren't committed to our own growth (and falling the fuck in love with ourselves), encountering a soul mate may prove elusive. We may meet someone with whom we feel an instant connection only to be reminded of the work we still have to do. Or we could be searching for someone to complete us (a paradox) only to discover that we contain the qualities within our own psyche we so desperately seek from another.

Let's say we do all this self-reflection and spiritual growth, and our soul collides with another that just seems to fit. What are the chances that that person has been making the effort to align themselves closer to their own truth? If and when we come together, can we each stay connected and evolving and dedicated to the trials and tribulations that come with letting love flourish? Do you believe that it is possible to find a kindred spirit and have your values and timing align? I do.

Just as we can experience more than one deep, long love in a lifetime, if we are lucky, we can meet more than one soul mate. I've encountered a few thus far. Sometimes they show up in the most unlikely places and forms—to teach us, love us, strip us bare, and leave us pondering our existence. It's all fodder for growth.

I may present an idealistic vision of love to strive for here, but remember that we are all humans and we are going to fuck up. It's in our nature. We just have to keep trying. It comes down to committing to love and all of its obstacles. I don't mean commitment to staying in an unhappy relationship or dynamic. I mean committing to showing up for love, committing to opening up to all the ways love expresses and exists. Love can break us open, make us face parts of ourselves we'd rather not look at, and transform us in the most beautifully unexpected ways. The more we expand our capacity for love in all forms—including love for community, family, friends, self, partner, nature, spirit—the more love we are ready to give and receive. I may not ever get to the bottom of what love is, but I am willing to die trying.

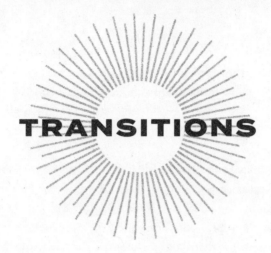

TRANSITIONS

As we move through life, we confront various rites of passage and what may appear to be obstacles in our path. I call them "transitions." These can include adolescence, adulthood, and aging; health issues; the loss or the death of a loved one; exploring sexual identity; gender transitioning; breakups, heartache, or divorce; a new residence or career; spiritual awakening; and more.

Facing any one of these life shifts, let alone multiple ones at once, can cause extreme unease, despair, and uncertainty, both for ourselves and for others in our lives. Staring into the abyss of the unknown is an awkward place to be. We may want to run away from these stages of our evolution because they are too complex to face.

As we transition, we are transforming and transcending, from one place to another. It's the in-between stage—also called *liminal space*—that tends to cause our minds the most trouble, when we, or another person, are neither here nor there, having begun the journey but not arrived at the conclusion. An elevator or escalator is a concrete example of liminal space. Or in the case of someone who is in the process of changing their sexual or gender identity, they are experiencing a death of or a goodbye to their old self and are in the process of integrating into a new form.

I envision liminal space as something like the life cycle of *Mechanitis polymnia* butterflies during their pupa, or chrysalis, stage. They have a protective chrome-like exoskeleton that provides shield and shelter as they transition from caterpillar to butterfly. It looks like a brilliant golden armor. Inside, they are going through a cellular dissolution of their previous form, literally turning into liquid goo. This stage of leaving one form to become another is called *metamorphosis*.

When I'm going through a life change, impatient for manifestation and resolution, it helps me to think of these butterflies suspended in their cocoons, waiting for a new existence to reveal itself. Within the discomfort and pain of whatever it is I am facing, keeping this visual in mind allows me to find beauty in the liminal space.

Other people may shun us as we are in the midst of a transition, especially when we need extra support and understanding. Have you ever felt uncomfortable with someone's sickness or outward grief? Not known what to say to someone who has new pronouns or publicly identifies with a different gender or sexuality expression than you are used to them having? Maybe a close friend or family member you thought was in a solid partnership is breaking up, and it's bringing up all sorts of mixed emotions you'd rather not feel about your own relationship. We often distance ourselves from the people and things that provoke dread in us only because we lack practice, skills, and the vocabulary with which to do so.

When we do something contrary to society's belief system, like transition our gender, divorce, or publicly grieve, it triggers fear in others. People don't always like it when we do the opposite of what they are used to; it may even cause them to feel angry or nervous. We could be challenging their idea of the status quo simply by our very existence, because we can't be placed into a neat little box. It may be difficult to remember at these points, but *what other people think of us is none of our business.*

We are all just trying to figure ourselves—and life—out. What if we allowed more space around the change process instead of forcing conclusions from ourselves and others? Is there room for us to explore amid the boxes our culture wants to put us into to make our identities more neat, tidy, and easy for people to understand? Sometimes we don't even know what box best describes where we are at right now.

What if we called the stage of figuring out what-the-what is happening to me/him/her/them/us *metamorphosis*? What if we didn't force ourselves or others to arrive at an end point before we or they were ready and instead allowed nature to take its course? With sexuality and gender identity in particular, we may feel pressure (and other people absolutely might push us) to define ourselves in a certain way, whereas transitioning in and of itself is a journey. None of it happens overnight, as much as we may want it to. There are so many opportunities for growth, acceptance, and miracles along the way if we can stay present with the process. As the poet Gwendolyn Brooks so eloquently put it:

Live not for battles won.
Live not for the-end-of-the-song.
Live in the along.

Easier said than done, I know. Especially when the journey of discovery itself can be so anxiety inducing and a struggle for us to explain to ourselves, let alone others.

Trans activist and journalist Ashlee Marie Preston told me that her

> highest points of personal growth have always been leaning into discomfort. . . . There are moments where I . . . have so many different things at play. I'm attracted to men, [though] not so much sexually, really. I have to be into the person, almost like a sapiosexual[36] . . . sometimes I can find a woman attractive. My ex-boyfriend was a trans man who was assigned female at birth. We had similar lived experiences. I didn't have to take on the labor of having to explain, and I also didn't have to apologize, because we understand that we're trying to figure all of this out and it's chaotic and crazy and fluid and ever changing.

Preston's experience shows just how fluid matters of gender and sexuality can be. Yet in so many ways, especially when it comes to sexuality and gender identity, we seem to be collectively stuck in binary thinking, all black and white with little or no nuance. Dr. Amy Weimer founded the cutting-edge UCLA Gender Health Program at the University of California, Los Angeles. The program offers comprehensive medical and surgical care to the transgender and gender-diverse community in Los Angeles and across the United States. As she puts it,

> When I was raised, there was no concept of having a gender identity other than male or female. People who identified as transgender still identified as strictly transgender male or transgender female. The new

_____

36 This term describes someone who is sexually aroused by and/or attracted to intelligence. Some who identify as sapiosexual care only about the other person's intellect, while others may also identify as heterosexual or within the LGBTQIA+ spectrum. Debate is ongoing as to whether sapiosexuality is an orientation or a fetish. As long as their object of desire has a big . . . brain.

construct—which is particularly embraced by younger people—[is] that there are plenty of people who fall outside of that binary, people who identify as not exclusively male or female. Those are what we call nonbinary identities. But within that, there are a lot of different identities that people might claim: two-spirit identities, gender fluid, agender. I think it's really important to hear from each person what their description of their gender is. It may evolve with time.

Everything and everyone—especially and including nature—is in a continuous state of flux. We count on love to stay forever, people to be with us forever, our bodies to stay the same, life and the world as we know it to be predictable, but nothing is a given. Change is scary, yet it is the only constant we can count on. Maybe what makes a transition even harder is our own anxiety getting in the way.

My friend Bill T. Jones is a choreographer, director, dancer, and author. He is the cofounder of the Bill T. Jones/Arnie Zane Dance Company and one of the most brilliant men I know. I've been privileged to see him rehearse, conduct pre-show rituals, and perform with his company on multiple occasions. Whenever I am filled with apprehension, I think of watching Bill backstage before a performance. As part of the warm-up exercise and blessing, he gathers his dancers in a circle, instructing them to shake off each limb as though flicking aside nerves or water. Toward the end, he tells them that whatever is left in their stomach (nerves, fear, butterflies) is "pixie dust." Is it possible that fear—not the kind we have when facing a threat, but the kind we experience when taking a healthy risk or making a change—might be the same thing as excitement?

Could we embrace something (a transition) that causes us and others distress? Could we notice our own and others' apprehension and choose to be brave and bold anyway? That old binary thinking tells us that an experience that looks or is supposed to be "bad" can't contain levity. Yet all these feelings can coexist, just as in pain there is discovery and in heartache there can be joy. In the midst of a relationship transition, for example, is a possibility to evolve our understanding of love and partnership, to learn new patterns. Grief and love are interlinked—have you ever been in the depths of heartache and felt comforted by endless tears? Or laughed aloud at a heavy moment? Whenever I can't help laughing while relaying terrible news, I think of Joni Mitchell singing, "Laughing and crying / You know it's the same release."

Life and humans are kinetic, not static. We are constantly changing, experiencing both losses and expansion. When it comes to aging and death—transitions that *every single human* will go through—it seems the entire Western culture, including the media, is built around avoiding it. As much as we are culturally uncomfortable speaking about sex, we *really* don't want to accept that we will all get older and eventually transition out of our bodies.

There is a prevalent social message that sex is for the young. If you've read this far, you know that sexuality is not only about penetration. As we evolve, so does our relationship with our bodies and sensuality. Regardless of our stage in life, most of us require touch and close relationships with other humans. As we get older, we may explore different methods of achieving physical connection; we may need more mental stimulation or more time to become aroused. If we are aging together with someone in a relationship, we may be transitioning from lust to love—or our sex may be hotter than ever.

In our youth-obsessed society, it may be impossible to believe that growing old and gaining wisdom were once celebrated. Although westerners have many fears about menopause and impotence signaling a decline of health, vitality, and sexuality, in other cultures (and in ancient ones) this was a time for increased prestige, power, and self-esteem. The crone, or wise older woman archetype, had powers of healing and intuition; she could connect more consciously to her spiritual and sexual energy. I was looking forward to turning forty from the time I was thirteen. I felt it was the age when I would officially become a woman, and I'm looking even more forward to being a superpowerful, magnetic sixty-year-old who is having the best sex of her life.

The following are some facts and thoughts on aging that can be applied however you identify. I'm using binary (male/female) language here, as the research that my conclusions were taken from was based on historical accounts and old models of sexual health and data. Remember, the medical system still has a lot of catching up to do when it comes to sexual and gender identity.

Menopause is a life transition that begins when people who menstruate stop having menstrual cycles. This is a process, not a single event. Over a two-to ten-year period, they will be dealing with sexuality and menopausal changes. It can begin between the ages of forty-eight and fifty-two but also on either side of this range. Perimenopause can begin in the thirties—this is not often talked about—and is *totally normal* if that is the way your body functions. A doctor can best advise if you are experiencing menopause or perimenopause.

During this time, as ovarian hormones decline, symptoms can include hot flashes, night sweats, depression, irritability, sleeplessness, concentration problems, mood swings, and breast tenderness. Also to look forward to (joking) are changes in the vagina, the progressive loss of pubic hair, and the lining of the vulva[37] becoming thinner and losing elasticity. This can cause pain, especially during intercourse. Here's where lubrication[38] becomes incredibly important. If it is legal in your area, a cannabis-based lube may do wonders.

Aging, no matter your gender, includes the difficult psychological task of accepting that there will be less time ahead, accompanied by undesired physiological changes. For postmenopausal women, there is also the acknowledgment that child-bearing years have come to an end. Want to know the silver lining of menopause? Women tend to experience the height of their sexuality around this time. As menstruation starts to diminish, libido may be stronger than ever. The famed actress, screenwriter, producer, playwright, and self-styled femme fatale Mae West apparently had multiple lovers and an endless lust for sex up until the day she died at eighty-seven.

The flip side of this is more common for men. Typically, around the same age as women are experiencing menopause, men are masturbating less, having less sexual fantasies, and experiencing more issues with erectile dysfunction, or ED. It is estimated that about 55 percent of fifty-five-year-old men have ED; after age seventy, about 70 percent of men; and so on. As men age, ejaculation doesn't occur each time they orgasm, and orgasm may not occur at all.

Culturally, male sexuality is linked to performance and intercourse. If performance requires an erection, aging plus the possibility of impotence equals terror. This is a masculinity paradigm we need to shatter, as it holds men to impossible ideals *and* denies them the ability to expand their experience of pleasure as they age. On top of the frustration and shame that accompanies ED and loss of sexual vitality, men often receive less than empathetic responses from heterosexual partners. Many women interpret a lack of erection as a lack of desire for them—or, worse, berate their partner when they may be at their lowest.

When it comes to pharmaceutically assisted erections, we enter into yet another example of medical hypocrisy around sexual health. (Another area for

---

37 The vulva is the visible, external part of cis-female anatomy. Often in society and casual conversation, this area of anatomy is referred to as the *vagina*, which is anatomically incorrect, the vagina being an internal canal where penetration can occur and babies may be birthed from.

38 If you are wondering why foreplay is imperative in heterosexual partnerships and hookups, know that it can take twenty to thirty minutes for a woman of any age to become naturally lubricated. Dr. Walter Brackelmanns and Dr. Wendy Cherry loved to talk about the "20/20 rule," meaning that it could take twenty minutes for a vagina to get wet, while a penis could become aroused in only twenty seconds. Talk about an orgasm gap!

science and medicine to improve upon, while we are at it: let's invent male birth control that actually works.) Did you know that the erection medication Viagra is covered by insurance while menstrual products are not? This double standard only increases the myth and expectation that sex is just about intercourse for men.

Although I've come across more than one company pushing "female Viagra" as a feminist (capitalist) miracle in a pill, I believe it to be a fallacy. Viagra prescribed for erectile function operates on a mechanical level, while a range of factors (hormones, mood, environment, et cetera) contribute to vaginal arousal, not the least of which is brain stimulation.

Aging and the anticipation of death are perhaps not enjoyable to ponder for most of us, but maybe they would be less intimidating if we had more positive messaging around the process. Perhaps we could collectively confront and accept these experiences as a healthy, natural part of being human. The more we fight against, resist, or ignore monumental life shifts, the more arduous they are to experience.

Maybe the most distressing part about aging, besides the physiological changes to our bodies, is that we become closer to our own mortality.

I used to be really freaked out about death, even though (or maybe because) over the course of my life I've lost a lot of people close to me. Some were friends my age taken suddenly, before reaching adulthood. Others, like the burlesque queens I befriended when they were in their seventies and eighties, slowly deteriorated at the end of long lives. All of these deaths broke my heart. But mortality overall remained a concept that I was unwilling to brave.

My ex-husband got really frustrated with me when we were meant to be jointly figuring out end-of-life planning. I refused to acknowledge, let alone discuss, pulling the plug; cremation versus being buried; organ donations; and beyond. There was no way I was going to think about him dying or that I would too one day. It was this huge, scary, unthinkable subject that seemed better to avoid.

I've known enough people suffering from terminal illnesses to witness the commonality of loved ones holding them back from death because they can't imagine life without them. Instead of helping someone by releasing and supporting them with love, we may become selfish, focused on how their absence is going to affect *us*. Often we are mourning someone before they are even gone—living in the future, thinking about our projected misfortune, instead of in the present, noticing their experience of this final transition. Even funerals are for the living, though they can be a beautiful celebration of the person who has passed.

Is it possible for us to become more at ease with death so that we can better attend its eventuality? My father's passing was my first inescapable, front-row view of death. It clarified for me the need to lean into transitions that cause the most anxiety and to develop grounding techniques with which to meet them. Or—and this might sound strange—to develop a practice for dying.

One night a few weeks before my father passed, I was visiting with him when he experienced a spiritual reckoning and realization that death was imminent. I'd seen this sort of thing in movies and read about it in books—where the person's life flashes before their eyes, they are visited by an angel of death, and they're filled with regret, longing, and fear—but I always thought it was a fictional device.

As he worried aloud over long-past transgressions and a lack of personal faith, he worked himself up into such a state of alarm that he struggled to breathe. Strangely, I was never calmer in my life. I don't know where it came from, but suddenly I knew to reassure him that he had been a good man, just a human, after all; that it wasn't time to die just yet; that he should try to breathe slowly; that there were angels surrounding him. Mind you, I wasn't raised with any religion and had never talked doctrine with my dad. It just seemed like he was needing something to hold on to as distress made his body even weaker. It was one of the last coherent conversations we had. He was admitted to the ICU that night as his oxygen levels dipped dangerously low.

With some distance now, I think about this moment and the analogy of being caught in a riptide in the ocean. In the chapter "Filling the Void," I talked about emotions being like waves: eventually they will pass, but it's hard to remember this when you are in the middle of painful ones.

The word for wave in Hawaiian is *nalu*. Nalu also implies a meditative state of being—to allow yourself to flow with what is. As the Hawaiian cultural leader and practitioner Lei Wann told me, **"People will say, 'I'm going to nalu with it,' meaning they accept what is in this moment even if they don't agree with it or it troubles them; they will ponder it instead of letting it overtake them."** Waves rise and crash and recede like emotions do, but we are not the sum of our waves. We are each surfers on our own oceans, riding the waves of our feelings until their power disperses.

Staring down death could feel like being held under by a wave or trying to swim against a riptide. If you panic and give in to the fear and struggle that arise, you come up against a heightened sense of mortality, causing even more terror. My friend the surfer and parking-lot philosopher Jean Paul "J. P." Marengo told me that

> getting sucked under by a wave is like, wow, man. It totally takes control of you and pushes you down under water. The normal reaction when you're getting rag-dolled and rattled by this wave is to fight back or to push against it. Actually the thing to do is to let it just take you, don't fight it, and reserve your oxygen. If you retaliate and push against it, you're using oxygen. If you get held under longer, you're going to be out of breath and risk whatever the circumstances [present], which could be drowning. It's one of those things you have to practice, and it's hard because you're not in control. So when you're not in control, you gotta let go and be calm in the chaos.

Many big-wave surfers—I'm talking about world-class athletes who are riding fifty- to one-hundred-foot waves—utilize breath work as part of their extensive training regimes, in preparation for the risk that comes along with their sport. Some practice holding their breath underwater while carrying rocks across a pool or the bottom of the ocean until they can't breathe anymore and need to come up for oxygen, achieving progressively longer times as they train. Even surfers who aren't necessarily riding big waves might practice holding their breath underwater for two or three waves in succession. The breathing techniques espoused by extreme athlete and author Wim Hof, nicknamed "the Iceman," are also extraordinarily popular among surfers and civilians alike.

Developing a conscious breath practice is not only potentially lifesaving but also has a hugely positive impact on every area of your life, from reducing stress to laying the foundation for having better orgasms and truly transcendent partnered sex.

On an average day we take roughly twenty thousand breaths. But unless we practice meditation or yoga regularly, chances are we are not aware of *how* we are breathing. When we get stressed, anxious, or upset, we often unconsciously constrict or hold our breath. We get so spun out in our minds that we may feel out of control or out of our body.

There are hundreds of breath exercises that can help calm our parasympathetic nervous system when this occurs and ground us back into our body. A simple one to practice is four-seven-eight breathing. Take an in-breath with your nose, filling up your belly and diaphragm for a count of four. As you breathe in, focus on where the breath is hitting in your body—you may even start to feel your spine elongate. Fill up completely with air as you count. At the top, hold your breath for a count of seven. Then slowly exhale, releasing the diaphragm down to the belly for a count of eight. And repeat.

In the midst of writing this chapter, I had to use four-seven-eight breathing when I had a panic attack after a pedicure appointment ended up causing me to have to get my left big toenail entirely removed. My personal biggest fears are doctors, needles, and tsunamis, so being told I was going to have several shots of lidocaine in my foot followed by the surgical removal of my nail sent me into a tailspin. Normally I would take antianxiety medication before any kind of surgery just to be able to have an anesthetic shot, but there wasn't time. I asked the doctor to let me sit in the room for fifteen minutes to calm myself down before the procedure. Then I called a friend, who reminded me that I was "the queen of breath work," so I'd better buck up and take my own advice. I did four-seven-eight breathing up to and during the entire procedure and managed to get through. My doctor even asked to give me a hug when she finished because she was so proud of me for facing my fear.

The Hawaiian word for breath is *hā*. If you take a deep breath in and then exhale while saying an extended "hā" (pronounced "haaaaaaaaaa"), you may feel a sense of calm come over you. It is believed (both in Hawaii and across the world by many) that *ha* helps you connect with your *mana*—your empowerment, mind, soul, spirit, the energy that lives inside you and is unique to you. If you practice yoga, you may have heard mana called "prana" or "qi." Lei Wann says that "the practice of hā can be used anytime. It comes into play when practicing hula [traditional dance and song]; and in *lua* [martial arts] you can be even more powerful using your breath against an opponent than with your physical anatomy. In *lomilomi* [Hawaiian massage technique] hā can bring things out of your body as a method of releasing, because as we know on a scientific level breath releases stress."

Breath work can even be used to grapple with death. Barbara Carrellas is a sex/life coach, the founder of Urban Tantra, and the author of several books on the topic. Urban Tantra is an approach to conscious sexuality that adapts and blends a wide variety of sacred sexuality practices, from tantra to BDSM. She uses breath work as a cardinal tool in tantric workshops as well as in helping people transition to the end of life. She explains the remarkable power of working with the breath:

In times of real deep sorrow or around tragic or violent events, we might do a dedicated kind of breath and energy orgasm. For instance, I led one for about a hundred gay men, many of whom were HIV-positive survivors of the epidemic and others who were younger and were not survivors. That was incredibly powerful for both the men who were not adults during the plague and equally or more so for the survivors who had been living with survivors' guilt and shame.

More recently, one of the founders of Urban Tantra, Catherine Carter, died of a brain tumor. She and I used to practice for death under massage tables where people were receiving erotic massages. We would breathe with them, hidden by the sheet that covered the table, and provide energy from below. When they had an orgasm or did the clinch-and-hold breath energy orgasm technique, we would take it and practice disappearing, dying, going away. I reminded her of that. I said to her, "Cath, we've practiced death a lot, you're really good at it." I think that I've explored death a lot through breath and energy orgasms. I don't know if any of us know how to die perfectly, though. I seriously doubt it.

Beyond helping calm us in moments of extreme transition, we can use breath work to heighten our awareness and experience altered states of consciousness. I try to maintain a kundalini Breath of Fire practice every morning to clear my mind and help me drop into my body. Breath of Fire is rapid, continuous, and rhythmic, done through the nostrils with the mouth closed, with an inhale and exhale of equal lengths and no pause in between. It sounds almost like a puppy panting. Though it can quickly bring me out of my spinning mind and into an exalted state, this is not a practice that is recommended if you are menstruating or pregnant.

I recommend trying a number of different breath techniques for different situations. I have mentioned a few above, and we will get more into breath exercises in the next chapter. Any type of breath work—whatever works for you—helps bring patience, calm, and grounding in the present. Try breathing fully in moments of fear, anxiety, or transitions; deep breathing can also be applied to all other aspects of overall wellness. It can alter our response to change and move us out of being rigid with how things are "supposed" to be. This allows us to give in and let go when we are experiencing things that are out of our control and overwhelming, like grief or heartbreak.

When we can find presence *in this very moment right now*, we can better meet our life with joy, seizing love wherever we can find it, even in times of great stress. Much of our fear is caused by anticipating the future, while anxiety can be induced by thinking about the past. Staying present is being *mindful*. Diana Winston is the director of mindfulness education at the UCLA Mindful Awareness Research Center, otherwise known as MARC. As she says, "Mindfulness is paying attention to our present-moment experiences with openness and curiosity and a willingness to be with what is. It's about living in the present moment, not lost in the past, not lost in the future, which is typically where our minds go. It's also where a lot of anxiety lies and a lot of grief, ruminations, fear. We're often in the present moment wishing it were a different present moment, right? So mindfulness is this invitation to right here and right now."

When I catch myself engaging in catastrophic thinking, I recall the title of one of my favorite books, *Be Here Now* by Ram Dass. Or in my updated idiom: *DON'T FUTURE FUCK*. By "future fuck" I mean you can drive yourself bananas going over and over all the possible outcomes of whatever situation you are worried about—usually before there actually is anything to worry about. Especially in a new relationship, this is important to remember. Stay present with what is and face what might be when you get there.

I'm not going to pull any punches here: there's a lot of opportunity for future-fuck thinking right now. We are collectively experiencing a massive transformation at this very moment, with climate change and disease upending the planet. With so much global uncertainty and suffering, it is more imperative than ever to find a grounded place to operate from in the midst of all this transition and upheaval. Mother Earth deserves our attention, urgently.

I mentioned earlier that one of my biggest fears is tsunamis. I live in California, which is subject to earthquakes, raging fires, and an ongoing drought. Since childhood I've had nightmares about the acceleration of climate change, and now it seems we have arrived at a point where the warnings are coming true. Yet I still have hope. Giving in to apocalyptic thinking only makes my fears worse and stops me from experiencing the magic and beauty of nature right here, right now.

I know it is a herculean effort to remain calm when things feel intense. I believe having mindful and spiritual practices is crucial as world issues spiral further into horror-plot zones and our thinking clouds up with overwhelm.

We need whatever tools we can develop (hope, love, faith, breath, joy, sex!) to meet and rise above the challenging days ahead. To stay focused on creating new systems as the old ones burn, we need to stay connected to the divine.

Developing a deep intimacy with yourself through a spiritual practice can provide you with the ability to gain higher perspectives through conscious emotional detachment. Being mindful or practicing meditation also allows us to detach enough to see beyond our own circumstances. There's something very powerful about prayer, meditation, and asking for help. Sometimes when I feel really lost, I will close my eyes, take a few deep breaths, and say the words (aloud or internally) "I surrender." Meaning, "I surrender my worries to something greater than myself," or "I give up this problem to a higher power for guidance." Often I will imagine a departed beloved ancestor holding me or their voice telling me it will be okay; other times I try to visualize being held by a special place in nature, like a favorite tree or the ocean.

As a child, my mother actively discouraged me from connecting with religious practice because of her own conflicted relationship to faith. She went to Catholic school in an oppressive, regressive, small-town environment and developed an intense antipathy toward the dogma of organized religion, to the point where she made me feel it was "unintelligent" to connect deeply with God. I literally begged to go to church or Hebrew school, and I read books on Buddhism when I was old enough to. All of which I felt ashamed to openly admit for years. Because I did not have formal religious education, my spiritual practice is taken from rituals and beliefs across a wide range of faiths. I have the freedom that my mother didn't, back in the 1950s, to reject or accept the dogma that works for *me*. So, for example, I will light candles in a shrine, temple, or church and pray, but I don't follow any scripture or believe that love is acceptable only between a man and a woman.

It is your right to create a personal definition of spirituality and spiritual growth that resonates with your heart and soul. Whether you were raised with religion or you reject dogma and organized structures, maybe we don't have to throw the baby out with the bathwater? As Ashlee Marie Preston told me, "Spirituality . . . for me is no singular doctrine or idea but a kaleidoscope of different traditions and ideals and entities and ideologies and streams of consciousness and intentionality. When I think of God, I don't think of this white guy up in the sky with Pantene-shiny hair. I think of God as all-encompassing. I don't think of God as gendered."

Cultivating a personal belief system is helpful in times of transitions and the darkest hours we face—those times when we are literally on our knees. Although I don't believe in regrets, I wish I had had the chance to create a foundational relationship with spirit earlier in life, as in the last few years it has been a gift to have that as a guiding course to channel through my art and sexuality.

I've had several off-line conversations with my friend Ramy Youssef about the role that faith plays in his work and personal life. And none of it is perfect. Nor does it have to be. Ramy says there is a concept in Islam "called the Ladder of Possibility, where God made angels, and humans, and jinn. Jinn are lower spirits. . . . There's a reason that we're slotted in the middle. This is definitive of what our existence is. If we [humans] were supposed to bat a perfect score, this middle section wouldn't exist. So it's kind of like life is about the struggle."

If you are facing a massive transition, it might be helpful to create your own ceremony of letting go. This could be as simple as writing a goodbye letter to someone (or to a period of your life, even to yourself!) and burning it, safely. You can even say aloud, "I release you/this" and visualize letting go, without regret or remorse. Easier said than done, and of course this person or part of your life will still occupy a part of your brain and heart, but the symbolic act of releasing sends an energetic signal that you are ready for a new chapter. I would urge you not to push yourself to do a letting-go ritual before you are ready! Or if others are pressuring you to. I am still salty that my ex-husband and college roommate shamed me into throwing away my favorite blanket from childhood when I was nineteen! On the other hand, if you are ready, such a ritual can be liberating. Upon delivering the first draft of this book, I burned a decade of my diaries to a crisp as an offering, a sacrifice, a release of the past. These journals contained my most intimate, embarrassing, enlightening, joyous, heartbreaking, erotic, and painful moments (some of which are immortalized in the pages you are reading). I know this may sound like a radical act, but carrying around those diaries for so many years felt like a load I needed to slough off as I entered a new phase of my life. It was so freeing to watch them burn!

The transitions we face in life are tremendous opportunities for spiritual growth and healing, a chance to gain a deeper understanding of our place in the world. I often think of a Hebrew phrase that I learned from Rabbi Denise Eger, who leads Congregation Kol Ami in West Hollywood: *tikkun olam*, or "heal the universe." Rabbi Eger is one of the first openly lesbian rabbis to work in the United States, and she was the first queer president of the

Central Conference of American Rabbis, the largest organization of rabbis in the world. I asked her if the phrase meant that every human being has a task to bring justice and healing to a broken world—and to ourselves along the way. As she explained to me,

> The mystics, the Kabbalists, of our tradition had a way to understand creation. You won't find this story in the Bible, but this is how they imagined it: that God sent out a great light and that light was to be contained in seven sacred vessels. But the light was so powerful and so beautiful that it shattered the vessels, sending the shards through the seven heavens down into what became the Earth. Those sparks of divine fire reside in each human's soul and in everything. . . . Even a table has sparks in it. Our job is to help uncover the sparks and to find those broken shards and put them back together. When we do that, in that task of healing and putting back together the brokenness of the universe, that's how we'll heal the world. We do that through acts of justice, acts of truth, acts of charity.

As I type these words, I am experiencing multiple transitions: moving, grieving, evolving, healing, and awakening—does it ever end? By the time you read this book, I will be undergoing another set of shifts, and you will, too. I recently got back on a surfboard for the first time since I was a teenager. I forgot how fun (and scary) it is to be out there, facing the possibility of getting barreled by a set or effortlessly gliding toward shore on a perfect wave. Although transitions are uneasy, they can inspire a breaking open that can be incredibly freeing.

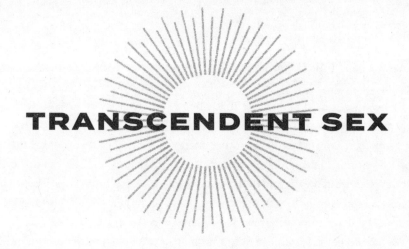

TRANSCENDENT SEX

Congratulations! Now that we've covered the foundational aspects of sex, health, and consciousness and looked at how they enhance every part of your life, you are ready for advanced-level education. Consider this chapter the pathway to harnessing the awesome power of your sexuality and achieving mind-blowing states of pleasure.

I have referenced a lot of hard data and scientific research in this book, which I think is important when it comes to grounding our understanding of sexuality. But there is another, more mysterious aspect to sex that is hard to quantify—the energetic, spiritual dimension. I normally keep my mystical beliefs around sexuality separate from the basic sex education we do at The Sex Ed, lest I get thrown under the bus by Dr. Jen Gunther (a gynecologist and writer who debunks myths and questionable advice offered by Internet "I do my own research" self-appointed doctors of sex). But at this point, with more than thirty years of background in the subject, what interests me most personally and professionally is the intersection of the practical and the divine.

I want to let you in on what I save for off-line conversations with some of my most open-minded intimates. Some of it might strike you as peak cringe woo-woo, but keep an open mind (and your ass will follow). While I may not be able to refer to controlled clinical studies here, I can point to anecdotal evidence and the ancient traditions of Taoism and tantra,[39] which contain

---

39 Tantra and Taoist philosophy have been widely misunderstood and misinterpreted by westerners and require a lifetime of study, so let me clarify that I am a mere student in these matters, not an expert.

functional and esoteric techniques that are applicable to twenty-first-century sex and beyond.

By now, we should all be clear that when I refer to "sex" or "sexuality," I do not mean for you to interpret these terms narrowly as penetration, orgasm, or genitalia. I consider sex and sexual energy to be potent forms of creativity and communication, which is expressed, on one plane, at the physical level. However, if mind, heart, and body are connected, we tap into the possibility of spiritual expression. This strengthens not only partnered sex but also how we channel (and are empowered by) sexual energy in our everyday life.

We have to get real and face things we may have avoided in the past in order to expand our capacity for cosmic orgasmic bliss. This means being clear on the ways in which we *use* sex—to fill a void, to self-soothe, to exploit, to escape, or for pleasure—and developing the discipline to heighten our sexual experiences. Clarity is called for not only with ourselves but in how we communicate with and even choose our sexual partners.

For example, if you are someone who desires sex with no commitment or strings attached, be up front with prospective partners (or pay a professional for transactional sex—at the very least, don't condemn it as an option if that ultimately is what you are seeking). Manipulation, emotional or otherwise, has no place in sex. If you are in a monogamous relationship and want to explore sex with other partners, have that difficult conversation with your significant other. Suppressing our desires only makes them grow stronger. If you ultimately want commitment, be intentional in how you approach your sex life. Being sex positive or liberated means honoring what is right for *you*, communicating that positively, and respecting others for where they are at, too.

Reframing the way we think about sex (and its awesome and amazing power) may even change the way you engage with dating. Mykki Blanco told me, "Once I knew that sex could be this intimate spiritual [experience], it's changed a lot. Now, when I hook up . . . it's not this transactional Grindr hookup. I hate hookup apps. If you're into spirituality, I think they're low frequency. I think that you are only going to get the worst transactional sex out of them. I think they're bad for your self-esteem. I think that [for] this journey of allowing intimacy to be this spiritual sex consciousness, it's okay to feel vulnerable and safe and really, really take your time."

No shade or disrespect if digital apps are your thing—again, as long as you are conscious or mindful of how you are interfacing with them and what you fundamentally desire. I also want to share that I receive so many questions about sex, love, and dating prefaced by "I should have it figured out by now" or "I know I'm a late bloomer"—as though any of us were given a guidebook or the agency to go on a sexual self-discovery journey in the first place! Wherever you are is *exactly where you should be.*

The act of reflecting upon and integrating overall consciousness and connectedness between our heart, mind, and sexuality is the first step. Too much work to self-reflect, you say? Don't worry, this chapter will introduce a breathing technique to bring yourself to orgasm, hands-free, and offer some simple tools to introduce into your current sexual repertoire.

But if you are willing to *go deeper* (you've picked up this book and read thus far, so I believe you can do it), I promise your life—and sex—will be elevated by doing the deep inner work. The great thing is, as we get older, wiser, and more practiced, our sexual life can improve. It's not the message we are receiving in the media (as we learned in the last chapter), but it *is* a reality that is not out of reach.

The moment of orgasm, like a forceful meditation, breathing technique, or mind-altering substance, can be *transcendent* far beyond what you may have experienced. I'm talking over and above the ecstasy of lust and release. In New Age circles, you may have heard the term *vibrations*, or *vibes*, before. As in "He/she/they/that house has bad vibes" or "Man, she's giving me strong vibrations." It's basically another word for energy, an impression someone or something gives off or you feel internally.

If we want to experience transcendent sex, we have to pay attention to the vibrations we give off and receive. I don't let people wear shoes in my house and am equally careful (after a lot of trial and error) with my sexual energy, because I want to protect the work I've done in order to get to this place. In my opinion, there is an energetic and chemical bond that is created via orgasm. Particularly so if you are on the receiving end of penetration. So for me, as a highly sensitive heterosexual leaning woman,[40] if I am taking in someone else's energy, I have to be purposeful with sex.

For many of us, this energetic and chemical bond can take a long time to dissipate after a penetrative encounter. Have you ever been fucked by someone you didn't really like, respect, or trust and feel fantastic in the moment but have a hard time shaking it off for weeks or months afterward? Kind of like a psychic letdown or postpartum crash? Totally normal and attributable to this

---

40 Although I believe labeling myself as such is using another outdated paradigm.

vibration or connection. You may laugh, but I often tell people to use sage smoke to energetically clear out their pussy, dick, or asshole as a method of resetting their sexual energy. I am not suggesting you hold a burning sage stick *this close* to your genitals, but you can let the smoke waft toward you from a safe distance while concentrating on letting go of other people's gunk and/or your own trauma.

Yoni is a Sanskrit word meaning "vagina or womb." A yoni steam is a steam bath for the vagina, usually prepared with medicinal or calming herbs and flowers; it is used to regulate menstruation and assist in pregnancy and post-partum health. You may have heard this referred to as "vaginal steaming" by contemporary white wellness leaders, but it is a practice that originated centuries ago in African, Asian, and Mayan indigenous cultures and is still widely utilized today. Yoni spas exist across the globe, and many specialize in reproductive health services. So far, I have mostly come across this practice marketed for people with vulvas, although I see no reason why it shouldn't be experienced by anyone, regardless of genitalia.

Yoni steaming can also be used as an energetic release. Indulging in them is not about perpetuating a myth that vaginas are unclean or smelly. Friendly reminder that our genitals are self-cleansing (with the aid of warm water and sometimes mild soap). Be careful of snake-oil products advertised to "cleanse" or "balance" the vagina (like douches), as using them can disrupt the natural vaginal pH balance. If you are interested in trying this practice, I urge you to seek a professional facilitator or a spa instead of doing it amateur style at home for the first time, as you run the risk of burning yourself.

It's odd that we spend so much time and money perfecting our skin and bodies, yet we rarely honor or nourish our genitals, let alone notice them outside of washing them, masturbating, or engaging in sexual activity. YouTube has thousands of hours of videos devoted to jade rollers and *gua sha* techniques for beautifying the face, based on well-established Asian health rituals. Yet we scoff at the concept of devoting ritualistic practice to our genitals. These are not 100 percent proven, medically backed methods for enhancing health, but neither is doing a "pore opening" facial or applying "hydrating night cream." If it makes you feel good about yourself (and your genitals) and is done safely, with a grain-of-salt mindset, why not?

Justin Simien, the multihyphenate creator of the incredible film and Netflix series *Dear White People*, among many other projects, has one of the sexiest brains I've ever been privileged to interview. "I think that sexual energy is really powerful, and we should treat it that way," he told me. "It's a very powerful energy, and it can get really mixed up with a lot of other things going on in our heads. I'm not celibate, but I've certainly fasted before both religiously and nonreligiously. And there is a clearing-out process that happens when you give something up that has a strong pull for you. You can untangle the motivations and the results and things that you just never could see before."

I think most of us are not tapped into the supreme power of our own sexual energy, and collectively (at least in the West) we are not intentional about how we direct it. The idea of sexual energy as life force is not a new one developed by green-smoothie-drinking California yogis. Its origins can be traced back thousands of years to diverse cultural and spiritual philosophies, including Taoism, which developed around the sixth century BC and is based on the writings of Lao Tzu in the Tao Te Ching.

I am paraphrasing what follows, and if you are an ancient Taoist scholar, I humble myself before you. Taoist principles include patience and being in divine harmony with the infinite force of nature. Central to the Taoist belief system is that life-force energy, or qi (a.k.a. chi, prana, shakti, mana, et cetera), is contained within us and should be in balance on an inner level *and* in our manifestations and engagement with others and the outer world. All of humanity and nature hold qi.

Before Lao Tzu solidified Taoist ideology in text, sometime during the Han dynasty (200 BC to AD 220), it was commonly understood that sex was linked to spirituality. It was also thought that sexual energy or exchange was capable of providing healing and transcendence—as well as the potential for the loss of life force. Taoists believed that bodily fluids (including semen) contained an essence (known as *jing*) critical to the life force, or qi.

The practice of restraining or delaying ejaculation comes from this philosophy of preserving life-force essence. As practitioners became experts in delayed or restrained gratification, it served their ability to channel the jing and use it to fortify and empower themselves. Hence the idea that sex did not have to conclude with a release. In Taoist texts devoted to sex and love, specific positions and techniques, including breath work and muscle exercises (we are going to try one together shortly), were recommended to achieve a high level of control over orgasm. These practices helped to harmonize mind, body, and spirit.

Later on in the twentieth century, the pioneering Western sex researchers William H. Masters and Virginia E. Johnson, known professionally as

Masters and Johnson, used a similar approach to treat premature ejaculation. Their method, published in 1970 as "the squeeze technique," helped prolong response to stimulation, increasing self-esteem, sexual confidence, and ejaculation time in study participants.

Now feels like a good time to check in with how our genitals are vibrating. Shall we?

In the introduction to this book I asked you to join me in a simple exercise to notice your genitals. We are going to practice it again, but this time we will introduce mindful awareness of our pelvic floor muscles and breath.

Everyone has a pelvic floor. These are a group of muscles and connective tissue that span the entire area of the pelvis. They support your internal reproductive organs and help control the anal sphincter, urethra, vaginal opening, and blood flow to the penis. Your pelvic floor regulates major bodily tasks, including urination, defecation, and sexual function.

To locate your pelvic floor, take a deep breath in and let it out. With your next inhale, squeeze the muscles you would use to stop your pee and hold them in. As you exhale, release those muscles. The muscles you just engaged make up your pelvic floor. Perhaps you've heard of Kegel exercises or been told to "practice your Kegels"? By tightening and releasing your pelvic floor muscles, you've just done a Kegel exercise.

Strengthening your pelvic floor muscles can aid in incontinence and intensify your orgasms. However, overexercising them or exercising them if you have underlying conditions (including being in a postpartum state) may be harmful. Check in with a trusted medical expert for what is right for you. For the following exercise, we won't be overdoing it.

Close your eyes and take a deep breath in. Hold your breath in for three counts and then slowly exhale, allowing your belly to fully release. Great. Now do it again twice more. Feeling settled? Now let's do it again, but as you exhale, bring your focus to your genitals. Observe any sensations there.

Now, with your eyes still closed, breathe in deeply, then exhale all the way down through your throat and into your chest, belly, and genitals. Do this slowly with me now, three times in a row. Is there any change in sensation? Whatever you are noticing, it is all good.

Let's build on that. Now, as you begin an in-breath, slowly tighten your pelvic floor muscles. Try not to clench your glutes while doing so. Breathe all the way in while holding these muscles. You may feel your belly tighten or your spine become more erect as you do.

Hold your breath for one beat at the top of your inhale and then slowly exhale, keeping your pelvic floor engaged until you release your breath at the very bottom, which should coincide with the exhale reaching your genitals. Try to release your pelvic muscles at the same time as you release your breath. Notice a tingling or warm sensation? Any difference at all? Try this a few more times, until you feel comfortable with syncing your breath and the muscles constricting and loosening.

Good work! The above breath pattern is stage one of orgasm breathing. I learned the basics of orgasm breathing from my friend and frequent The Sex Ed contributor Courtney Avery. Courtney, who has a master's degree in public health, is an E-RYT 200–certified yoga instructor and a birth doula. As she says,

> I like to teach a form of this practice that is easy for everyone to digest. It pulls energy from the base of your pelvis, where your sexual energy sits, up through the rest of your energy centers along the spine, filling you with life force. The benefit of this form of breath is that you will work the physical muscles of the pelvic floor while bringing the rest of the body into the exercise physically and energetically. Like any breath work technique, it focuses your mind on the breath and the physical body [because] concentrat[ing] the mind on something tangible [helps you] to reach a meditative or orgasmic state. The more you practice meditation, the more you train your brain to come into an orgasmic state. When you add the physical muscles and breath (energy) work into your sex life, magic happens. The potential to bring yourself into an orgasm with only the breath and muscle engagement becomes possible!

The first time Courtney taught me the fundamentals of orgasm breathing, I didn't believe it was possible to breathe myself to climax—and I expected it to happen quickly, after about fifteen breaths. Having patience with yourself is key for this exercise. Whether it takes you minutes, hours, days, or months, don't be like me and beat yourself up for not nailing it right away. Of course, practice makes perfect, so I set the mood to get serious about syncing my breath and pelvic floor engagement, with the intention of orgasming. I lit candles, took a bath, coordinated a romantic evening for myself, and got to work. It took a lot more than fifteen breaths, but eventually I got there. AND HOLY WOW!

As a fan of breath work's mind- and body-altering benefits, I have now experimented with various methods to bring myself to orgasm, without the aid of a partner or sex toy. Let me tell you, learning to incorporate mindful breathing into solo or partnered sex is a game changer.

Once I learned to breathe my way to orgasm, I became obsessed with teaching it to others. A few years after learning this technique, my partner at the time and I were on vacation in Mexico. We started each day practicing kundalini yoga together. He was not invested in spirituality, but he loved me and liked yoga as a form of exercise, so I convinced him to try kundalini. He couldn't believe how amazing the kundalini Breath of Fire and use of pelvic muscle control made him feel. Even better, our sex was more connected, culminating in intense climaxes—I even came close to blacking out after a cervical orgasm.

So imagine if you have two (or more) people who understand and are expanding their breathing, meditation, and muscle control practices—now we have the essential ingredients for transcendent sex. Once we expand our consciousness beyond seeing sex as strictly penetrative or orgasm based, we find the sacredness in it. Slowing down the process helps us move beyond instant gratification and into deeper intimacy and soul connection. Sacred sex can include touching, eye gazing, licking, and, yes, even breathing. Moving our sexual energy from the base of the pelvic floor up the spinal column is also the basis for much of what we (somewhat mistakenly) think of as tantric sex.

A few myths and realities about tantra:

1. Tantra is not a sex act. The Sanskrit word *tantra* (loosely translated as "to weave" or "weaving together") refers to a combination of Hindu and Buddhist traditions and a philosophy that emerged around AD 600 (give or take a couple hundred years). Tantra can include the use of mantras, devotional prayer, meditation, and rituals as well as a belief system.

2. It is impossible to give a sound bite or universally accepted definition of tantra.

3. In its long history, tantra's association with sex is a relatively recent development.

4. Applying classical tantric practice to sex can be likened to becoming mindful about sex, to an awareness that sex is an energy rather than

an activity. Tantric sex could be seen as weaving together the divine, or your consciousness, with the physical.

5. People who study tantra in the classical sense may work on their own pelvic floor exercises, breathing, meditation, and spiritual practice for many years before they partner with another person. This partner should be equally aligned within their own system of studies.

I am being nitpicky here about how the word *tantra* is used—kind of like how it drives me bananas when people refer to mass-produced fashion as *couture*. Whether it be exquisitely crafted hand-sewn clothing or a devotional practice of spirituality and sex, these rarefied labels take time, energy, patience, and skill to earn. That said, you can 100 percent integrate the philosophy of tantra into the bedroom without devoting a lifetime to studying it. It is really about the discipline of moving sex into the realm of your heart and consciousness. Which is why I love what Barbara Carrellas teaches through her books and workshop, Urban Tantra. She does a great job of incorporating tantric ideology into everything from fetish use to ecosexuality.[41]

Barbara broke down her relationship to tantra for me as such:

Tantra for me is a spiritual practice that says that we can have divine connection with something much bigger than ourselves, and spiritual wisdom, by going into everything on this earth completely and totally. Simply by going completely into what life gives us, every day, with total consciousness of commitment, you can reach spiritual realization, and you can do that with just about anything. You could walk the dog tantrically. You could do the dishes tantrically.

However, unsurprisingly, a whole lot of people like to do sex tantrically. Sex is something that they're deeply committed to going into completely. People often ask me, "Why is it all about the sex?" In fact, tantra isn't all about the sex. There's so many different

---

41 Codified by a new wave of radically sex-positive thought leaders (Annie Sprinkle chief among them), ecosexuality uniquely factors the natural world around us within human practices of sex and sexuality. This can look like anything from taking greater environmental responsibility when discarding used contraceptives, menstruation products, and sex toys to engaging sexually with plants, soil, stars, the moon, and/or bodies of water, with celebrating the stimulating effects of sex within nature falling somewhere in between.

schools and branches and lineages of tantra—many of which are still untranslated, hidden, [passed down through] oral tradition only, and exist [only] in the Far East—that we've never heard of. However, because it's a spiritual practice that says that sex is one of the ways that you can find spiritual truth, it is embraced by people who have been shamed or made wrong by other religions that are sex negative. So it's not surprising that in the West, when people say "tantra," most everyone thinks they are talking exclusively about an Eastern meditative form of sexuality.

When it comes to sex, essential to both tantric and Taoist philosophy are the notions that our sexuality and spirituality are intrinsically linked and that we can conserve, build, and discipline our use of sexual energy. I believe that we need to integrate and evolve our relationship between sex and spirituality or religious beliefs. So much of how we first learn about our bodies and desires comes from religious or cultural upbringing, and there is often a great deal of shame and judgment attached to adhering to strict dogma. If you were raised with any kind of religion or your parents were (or their parents and so on), most likely it had a huge impact on your views of sex and sexuality.

You may have been taught that being anything other than heterosexual was "wrong," according to the doctrine of your faith or that sex outside of marriage or even masturbation was a sin. You might have been brought up in "purity culture" and pledged your virginal innocence and devotion to Daddy until becoming betrothed to another man. If we are to align and reconcile our sexuality with our spirituality (or any higher power we subscribe to), we have to be able to develop a personal relationship to both. Faith and sex don't have to be mutually exclusive.

Brenda Marie Davies, host of the "sex-positive free-thinking Christian" YouTube channel God Is Grey, was raised with that separation between sex and faith. The author and podcaster grew up in a Roman Catholic home with a father who read her Bible bedtime stories. "God and my sexuality became powerful forces in my life, wholly separate from one another," she told me. "In my experience, the church has a disparate obsession with sexuality that's simply not mirrored in God's word. If I'd been permitted to read the Bible on my own, I'd have never gleaned sexual shame. I'd understand that God is love, that the Divine pulses through everything, including our loins." Although I'm no religious scholar, it would seem to me that faith is highly individual, as is our sexuality. Thus it's up to each of us to interpret and apply doctrine that allows for the most expansive experience of both.

Sahar Pirzada, who holds a master's in social work, is an organizer and educator focused on providing culturally sensitive sex education to Muslim communities across the United States. "I identify as a person of faith," Sahar says, "but I also identify as someone who is sex positive." As she put it,

> During the time of the Prophet [Muhammad], peace be upon him, people used to talk about sex pretty openly and ask really explicit questions about sexual activity. . . . If someone is a person of faith that's practicing their faith, I wouldn't imagine that they necessarily would be uncomfortable with talking about sex. There's a diversity in the community even where [in] certain communal spaces sex is openly talked about. And it's an intergenerational thing as well, where grandmothers and mothers and their kids will talk about sex and share tips. But they could still be very [much] practicing in their faith and adher[ing] to their faith values, and it's not necessarily seen as a contradictory thing.

Faith can assist as we transcend and surrender to love and pleasure. A practice of self-realization or fulfillment of your highest potential includes the potential for higher levels of energy exchange and pleasure during sex.

What we may consider disparate practices (for example, breath work and kink) can bring about altered states of consciousness when integrated with sexual activity. Experiencing subspace during bondage, for example, is a type of out-of-body transcendence. There are many IRL and virtual communities devoted to sacred kink or spiritual BDSM. In fact, one can say that this is a great example of integrating one's experience of their spirituality with their sexuality.

Barbara Carrellas told me that her parents

> attempted to raise me Catholic, and after an incredibly disillusioning, disappointing spiritual nonexperience at my first Holy Communion, I was extremely upset and feeling very betrayed because all the expectations I had for first Holy Communion, the way the nuns described first Holy Communion, was nothing short of a cosmic orgasm with God. And needless to say, it didn't happen [that way] in our little local parish.

So I went out and climbed my favorite tree and wrapped my seven-year-old legs around it and cried. The combination of emotion and bereftness and the scratchiness of the tree and the sexiness of the tree, I just went into this expanded orgasmic—although I didn't know the word or the concept at the time—state where all I could feel was something holding me and telling me, "It's going to be okay. There's something better." It was a profound energy orgasm that provided all the feels that I had been hoping to have at first Holy Communion earlier that day.

Speaking of fucking trees, I remember being stoned with a friend in Boston during high school and sitting outside under the stars as she waxed poetic about wanting to be "fucked by the moon." It was a sparkly crescent sliver, and I couldn't grasp, at the time, what the hell she was talking about. But much later, even before I knew the term *ecosexuality*, I realized that it was possible to have a direct erotic connection to nature simply by being in harmony with the qi of Mother Earth. I love to sit on a rock or a cliff at the edge of the sea and just open my legs up and receive the ocean's power into my vulva—not literally but metaphysically. I definitely feel that energy empowers me. Hey, don't knock it till you try it!

A side note here about using mind-altering substances to achieve transcendence. There is value in plant medicines, to be certain, but I would caution that relying on any kind of substances (natural or synthetic) is a little like looking out the window but not getting out the door. We need to do the diligent work of aligning our mind, body, and soul if we want to raise our vibration around sex, health, and consciousness.

Pleasure is essential as each of us faces another decade of political, social, personal, and climatic change. Wherever and however you can experience cosmic orgasms and ecstatic rapture—whether you find these in nature, sexual intimacy, breath work, fetish play, masturbation, maybe even meditation—we especially need these practices in order to meet the challenging days ahead.

The more we nurture a connection between sex and spirit, the more we see others as full human beings rather than mere objects of lust. The more intimacy we share, the more transcendent sex becomes a reality. As we rise above and question what has been, as old systems burn, we can create new ones that work for *us*, as long as we stay connected to our hearts and to the divine.

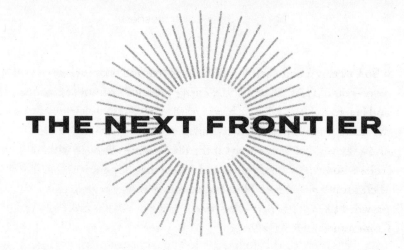

THE NEXT FRONTIER

My father used to say that back in the day, when it came to making Hollywood movies, films drew from only about seven story lines: "boy meets girl, boy loses girl, boy wins girl back"; "man and beast"; "man versus world"; "man versus machine"; and so on. Today, we see endless variables of these plotlines, but very few films break out of the basic formulas.

Similarly, most sexual activities, even those you might find outlandish or niche, have been practiced for centuries in some form or another. Today we may have updated our collective old story lines around sex with newer language, technology, and nuance, but are they all that much different from the stories people have been telling for centuries?

In AD 8, the Roman poet Ovid's poem *Metamorphoses* immortalized the tale of a sculptor, Pygmalion, who falls in love with a statue he's created in the shape of a woman. Pygmalion so desires his inanimate object of lust that she eventually becomes living flesh and his consort. Could Ovid have foreseen today's advanced sex dolls, whose robotic heads use cloud-based interactive artificial intelligence to "dirty talk" to your specifications? Or their temperature-controlled silicone vagina and anus orifices, designed to mimic the warmth of human ones?

The vertiginous heels worn by strippers today are the descendants of sixteenth-century chopines, high platform shoes worn by Venetian courtesans to protect their feet and dresses from mud and floodwater. In the eighteenth century, the nobleman, philosopher, and writer the Marquis de Sade was publishing erotic works that celebrated what were later termed "sadist" activities. Twenty-first-century BDSM involves (let's hope) more communication, consent, and boundaries than when de Sade was beating his housemaid and paying sex workers to participate in orgies.

So what is the next frontier? What will we value when it comes to sex? I believe it to be less about introducing new acts (you'll find that someone will have been there, done that previously, if you research long enough) and more about building frameworks that expand our understanding and experience of sexuality: *fluidity*, *intimacy*, *vulnerability*, *consciousness*, and *compassion*.

In the introduction to this book, I said that one of the biggest challenges we face on our sexual journey is to let go of what we *think* we know, like, or believe about sex. Let's broaden that to include letting go of assumptions around love, intimacy, relationships, and gender.

Here are some questions to consider as we enter the next frontier:

- How much of the way you move through life and your relationships is based on social codes, family expectations, and conditioning?

- Are your biases and fears holding you back from the process of exploration?

- Are you really being your authentic self?

- What are the relationship structures that best suit you?

- What do sexual freedom, expanded consciousness, and liberation from the old normal look like to you?

- Are you following your heart?

We need to decolonize our minds in order to set ourselves free. Many of us stop ourselves from embracing pleasure because we are stuck in a box of assumptions and practices born from a broken structure (the old normal). We may worry about what other people (friends, family, larger community) will think or how they may judge us if we reveal our true desires. The more we dig through our internalized shame, patterns, and stories and the more we define our own new normal, the more we are able to accept and love ourselves—and the more we are able to accept and love others. When we truthfully align our sexuality and consciousness, we create space for endless discovery.

I used to be the first to let insecurity and shame get the better of me, whether by resisting new things or being afraid to express vulnerability. Lately, though, I've been leaning into my trepidation as an opportunity to experience more pleasure. While I am far from perfect in this process, I try to notice, when hesitation arises, if it is simply part of the old conditioning. If it seems like it is attached to a story that doesn't belong to me, I try to stay open. I find myself attracted to all genders; what I am drawn to is an individual's mind and soul. Yet I was brought up in a (mostly) heteronormative social structure, and I fall in love and partner primarily with heterosexual men. So where does that leave these feelings? Does this mean I am queer *and* heteronormative? That I am a sapiosexual? Instead of attempting to define these answers, I try to stay fluid within what remains unexplored territory. Who knows what will happen in the future?

I want to offer a final exercise as we reach this last chapter together, one to help you begin shaping *your* next frontier. *I challenge you to challenge yourself* outside your comfort zone by building something new into your routine. Something that makes you genuinely happy, something that you've always wanted to try. Something that might make you a little afraid (in a healthy, good way) because you may not be good at it. Something you may have always held yourself back from trying for fear of failing. It might be drawing, dancing, singing, learning a new language or a musical instrument, practicing martial arts, or anything else you are curious about. Approach whatever this is with as much of a childlike mindset as possible. Try to practice whatever it is you choose for a set amount of time per day or week, setting a small goal for yourself and later expanding the time you dedicate to it gradually. For example, if you are learning to sing, begin by committing to fifteen minutes a day of singing. It's best to have realistic time expectations and then apply discipline to maintaining the practice. Stick with it and try to be lighthearted with the experience—this is something that is meant to bring you joy!

In the past year, I've been relearning how to surf, after not having been on a surfboard since I was fourteen. I have a healthy respect for the power of the ocean and more phobias (sharks, giant waves) than I did when I was a teenager. I am humbled by my lack of knowledge and skill as a new surfer (in surf slang, a "kook"). It's both terrifying and thrilling to be in a state of embracing the unknown, unsure whether I will wipe out or be stoked carving a glassy wave.

Fear of looking or sounding bad, of doing something "wrong" or not being "good" at something, is often what holds us back from reaching new heights of gratification. Generally, this anxiety surrounding a new situation or experience is way worse than the reality. Swap out surfing for having an uncomfortable but necessary conversation with a partner or introducing a potentially awkward new sex act into your repetoire, and you catch my drift. Our inner critic gets the best of us. We might feel we aren't worthy or that our sexual performance will fall flat. We overthink things instead of tuning in to our body and intuition—and remembering that sex is supposed to be fun! That it is, if we can just let go and enjoy it, whether or not we orgasm.

I literally have nightmares about trying to paddle out when the water is murky during shark season. In these dreams, a set of twenty-foot-plus waves is coming in. I have no choice but to head straight into the liquid walls. If I turn back, I'll be pummeled by white water. And the more I waver, the more likely I am to miss my opportunity to make it over to the other side before the next one comes. If I commit to the experience and push past the fear, my adrenaline and endorphins pump me up, and I feel fucking amazing! Kind of like someone experiencing an orgasmic sensation for the first time.

Today I was in the water with a pro surfer friend who has been giving me lessons. As we sat in the lineup watching sets (of waves), we traded off talking about each of our areas of expertise. He showed me how to read the waves—to tell which ones were breaking left, which were breaking right, and which were closing out—to help me better understand which ones to catch and at what speed I should be paddling to catch them.

In between, we talked about sex and romance. Seeing his expressions change as I told him why, for example, heterosexual men may enjoy being anally penetrated by their partner (because it stimulates the prostate, the equivalent of the G-spot for those with a penis) was as enjoyable for me as riding a wave.

At first, he was absolutely turned off by the suggestion of anal play. Surfing tends to the heteronormative, and though it is possibly the most "fluid" sport, historically, the culture surrounding it is less so. I suppose you could say this about most professional sports. Athletics is one of many areas where hetero-masculine "prowess" is most celebrated. The Roman gladiators who proved their skill in violent one-on-one combat before enthusiastic audiences in the colosseums were considered the most virile or fuckable. I remember as a teenager when NBA player Dennis Rodman was at the height of his Chicago Bulls fame. He was routinely in the headlines for dressing in drag and going to gay bars. Whether he was doing it as a publicity stunt to promote his memoir *Bad as I Wanna Be* or being his authentic self, Rodman challenged the NBA's largely (publicly at least) heteronormative fan base around gender and sexuality. Though times are changing, with more queer players coming out across different sports categories, they are still a small minority.

For many heterosexual men, the concept of ass play is taboo and considered effeminate. But why is this? Because if you receive pleasure from someone through this orifice, it denotes a certain sexual orientation? Why would you cut yourself off from the possibility that it could blow your mind? What if you convinced yourself that you only liked vanilla ice cream, but you had never tried chocolate because it was too "weird," and then one day you had some and realized you'd been missing out on something delicious for years? Prostate massage and anal play, incorporated into solo sex or with a partner, often allows for more powerful orgasms. Some men experience longer, harder erections with prostate massage and even their first multiple orgasms. At any age or time in your life, challenging yourself to look at something from a different perspective can unlock wonders. This is why I believe in keeping an open mind and staying receptive to your own fluidity.

When it comes to the way we collectively consider the spectrum of sexuality and gender, we should leave a lot of space for fluidity. In our old normal, adhering to strict patriarchal ideals of "masculine" and "feminine" often repressed or oppressed us, caused us to engage in toxic behavior, or made us the target for abuse. Some people shy away from potentially ultraorgasmic sex acts because they consider them to be "unmasculine." Embodying a more flexible mindset, along with a better understanding of the principles of yin (what has traditionally been known as feminine, receptive, passive) and yang (known as masculine, active, strong) energies might help us move past this old-fashioned thinking.

Regardless of your gender, sexuality, or whether you identify with the binary or nonbinary, we all contain aspects of yin and yang. Have you ever seen the symbol for yin and yang? It is a circle divided into two halves by a curved line. One half of the circle is black (yin) with a dot of white; the other half is white (yang) with a dot of black. It represents the duality and balance of nature, of the universe, of energies in constant flow and harmony.

When we are in a more fluid state, we can tap into and redirect our yin-yang energies, leading to enhanced sexual, personal, and even professional results. In 2015 I was studying tae kwon do in Los Angeles with Master Kim, who previously competed internationally, winning the gold medal while representing the US at the World Taekwondo Games (previously known by the unfortunate acronym "WTF") in Korea. Master Kim was teaching me tai chi as part of my training, explaining how to redirect yang (aggressive) with yin (passive) energy.

He told me that when he and his wife argue, he utilizes yin in order to resolve things smoothly and effectively instead of meeting her anger with yang energy.

Yang is not "better" than yin, nor do we need to ascribe gender to either. It is not "feminine" to cry or be vulnerable, just as it is not "masculine" to build a house. These modes of thinking are outdated, especially in the present, as AI technology is pushing us even further beyond binary thinking.

I talked to futurist philosopher Gray Scott about what he thinks our mainstream nonbinary future could look like. He told me,

> We're breaking apart that fifties nuclear-family idea of the mother, the father, and the kids. There are people that want to be in relationships with three people. There are people who don't identify as male or female. The portal that we're going through is leading us into a world where you can be anything you want in the digital landscape, once we create [mass] VR [virtual reality] and we're able to bilocate in two different places—meaning that we have our physical body in the real world and we have our avatar consciousness in the digital world. You're going to have a choice of identity in that digital world over not just your body but your sexuality and how you're presented to other people emotionally, psychologically.
>
> I'm going to paint a picture for you of, let's say, 2035. Everyone has either some sort of headgear or glasses that are augmented. So whenever you're looking out in the world, you're seeing the real world, but you're also seeing an overlay of digital information and animation laid on top. I can set a parameter so that everyone in the world looks like dragons if I want to. I can set my parameters for other people so that when they see me, they're forced to see me the way I want to be seen. So I can be a woman, I can be a dragon, I can be a robot. That is the world we're headed toward. Where the perceptual computing future gives you the choice to . . . alter not just your face but your body and what you represent to the outside world.
>
> So that brings up a lot of questions of continuity of psychology, continuity of body, continuity of sexuality. Am I female in the virtual world, but in the real world, when we take the glasses off, am I male? We're just looking at a future that is much more complex, [and] I think a lot of people are going to have a problem dealing with that complexity.

If this complex future is already upon us, we'd better get comfortable with fluidity, stat. A nonbinary reality has already existed since the dawn of time, both among humans and in the animal kingdom. For example, it is male seahorses, not females, who get pregnant and give birth to offspring. In many Native American and Pacific Islander cultures, third-gender persons, or those who ascribe to identities outside of what on the surface we have labeled "masculine" or "feminine," have been known by many different names, among them "two spirit," *fakaleitī*, and *māhū*. Such people have existed since long before contemporary language included nomenclature like *transgender*, *transmasculine*, *nonbinary*, *agender*, *transfeminine*, et cetera.

Hinaleimoana Kwai Kong Wong-Kalu, also known as Kumu Hina, is Kanaka, or Native Hawaiian. She is known for her work as a *kumu hula* (teacher of hula) and as a filmmaker, artist, activist, and community leader. She herself is acknowledged by some in her community as māhū, one who possesses the *mana* (power) of duality in life, the mana of both *kāne* (male) and *wahine* (female) in her daily experience. Kumu Hina also maintains a longstanding history of advocacy for the concepts of māhū and *aikāne* (a term for intimate relationships between the same gender) in her homeland of Hawaii.

As Kuma Hina explained to me,

> *Māhū* is the term that applies to an individual that possesses an element of both male and female, be it emotionally, mentally, [and/or] spiritually, as well as physically. Māhū I do not believe should be characterized as solely exclusive of one or another of the elements that I've just mentioned. . . .
>
> It is my understanding of the culture that I come from that indeed we are physical beings, but we come from a background and an understanding of mental, emotional, and spiritual groundings and understandings as well. My personal thought is that everyone is different, male, female, and māhū. So the subjective question is: Māhū, is it a gender identity? It is and it isn't; it's far more than just a sexual or a gender identity.
>
> I challenge you to look beyond the Western concept of masculine and feminine. What is masculine and feminine? [Say that] by Western standards you see a man [who is] extremely masculine, and he's very muscular, his features are what, in Western eyes, [you] would look at as very masculine. And then you see a biological

female who has much of the same aspects to her—strong jawline and facial features, larger bones, big hands, big feet—and somebody might be able to say, "Oh, that individual has masculine features." I don't believe that Polynesian culture comes from this kind of understanding where you delineate the masculine or what they perceive as masculine and feminine. . . .

I believe that some of the world's worst problems stem from people who cannot embrace all that their mind, their heart, and their spirit embraces. It's either too afraid, or it's too persecuted, or it's too uncomfortable for all of those individuals . . . and they end up engaging in very, very hurtful and destructive behaviors.

If and when we label certain emotions or actions as "feminine" (such as vulnerability or crying), we deny people who are biologically born as or identify as male from tapping into those emotions and nurturing their own growth. This repression forces those emotions underneath the surface. And then they get expressed as anger, violence, or fear instead of being processed and synthesized in a healthy way, through the lens of each person's individual experiences, spirituality, and heart.

Cultivating more vulnerability and intimacy is essential in the next frontier, within both our intimate and our nonsexual relationships. We cannot expect our primary partner or lover to be everything to us, nor we to them. It is crucial that we nurture other relationships that provide support, comfort, and companionship. To require our significant other, or any individual, to simultaneously play lover, coach, friend, parent, therapist, healer, and beyond is unrealistic. Yet we are culturally conditioned to desire all this and more from them. When we foster intimacy within a close group of confidants and community, we put less pressure on our partner to live up to the role of a fantasy superhero who can fulfill every need.

With regard to fostering intimacy, we are challenged by the current technological landscape, in which we are, as Sherry Turkle put it, "connected, but alone." If AI is at the forefront of how we are currently intimate and vulnerable with one another, I have some real concerns. For example, think about who is building the mass consumer technology we use daily and take for granted, like Instagram, Amazon, Google, fertility and dating apps, even facial recognition software. We readily submit our most personal information to these apps: who we love, who we fuck, our sexual and gender identities, when we bleed and ovulate, our moods, our physical features, our DNA sequencing, and maybe soon even our brains? All of these things that make us human. How valuable is this data? What does it mean that 90 percent of the people who create the technology we rely on are cis-het (read: straight) white men? How does that affect the way we interact with these tools and with one another? If we don't have a diverse group of people creating the products we depend on, how accurately will these products reflect the diversity of our experiences? And where do compassion, consciousness, and love fit into the equation?

I asked Stephanie Dinkins, associate professor of art at Stony Brook University and a world-renowned transmedia artist who creates platforms for dialogue about AI, whether she thought we were moving away from or toward intimacy in our interpersonal relationships. "I feel at the moment like we're disconnecting," she said.

> People are growing further apart. How do we make something that pulls us together, that becomes a partnership or sharing, rather than something that allows us to go off in our own corners and barely be together? Or the way that we're often together now, when people are together in the same space physically, but mentally, they're somewhere else? They're on their phones, they're not really in the same space and place at the same time. What would be the thing that brings us back mentally, consciously, into the same space?
>
> One of the things that I've recognized in also talking to people about AI, and making entities that one can talk to and look at and touch, is that people are looking for certain kinds of acceptance through these entities. That's what we're not getting from each other. I want to say we need to build an app that helps us to understand how to be intimate again, which is crazy, right? But how do we put it down? How do we make that space?
>
> I do think that love is super central to the idea of AI and it coming into being in a way that helps humans be more human. Recently, I was on a panel where there was a woman who was talking about what might save us in AI is this idea of unconditional love. If we can program the idea of unconditional love into our AI, we might be safe from that AI.

It's not just people like me and Professor Dinkins who are thinking about where love and consciousness fit into AI and VR. Top tech titans like Mark

Zuckerberg, as well as the US military, are also invested in this space, or they wouldn't be hiring people like William Barry, a leading AI ethicist, robotics communication specialist, and philosophy educator. Dr. Barry was a visiting professor at the US Military Academy at West Point and, as of 2021, serves as a subject matter expert in emerging technologies for the US Department of Defense. In 2017, while he was teaching at Notre Dame de Namur University in Belmont, California, a robot named BINA48 became the first-ever AI-equipped humanoid robot to complete a college course: Dr. Barry's Philosophy of Love class. Here's where things get even more sci-fi: BINA48 was born from a love story between an entrepreneur named Martine Rothblatt and her wife, Bina Aspen Rothblatt.

Martine Rothblatt is a tycoon, really— she created SiriusXM Satellite Radio and founded a biopharmaceutical company that provides organs for transplant. She is also a lawyer, philosopher, and transgender rights advocate. The accomplishments of her wife, Bina Aspen Rothblatt, include cofounding SiriusXM, United Therapeutics Corporation, Lung Biotechnology PBC, and the online World Against Racism Museum. She is also the cocreator of and inspiration for BINA48.

Together, Martine and Bina founded the Terasem Movement Foundation, whose mission is to promote geoethical use of nanotechnology for human life extension. The Terasem Movement Foundation supports scientific research and development in the areas of cryogenics, biotechnology, and cyberconsciousness. Quite a mouthful, huh? Stay with me, I promise this is related to love and consciousness.

I wanted to know more about BINA48's origin story, so I contacted Bruce Duncan, the managing director of Terasem. Bruce told me,

> Martine Rothblatt and Bina Aspen, being a couple in love, want to be in love together forever. It's the core motivation, so how would you do that? Once you're dead, you're dead, biologically speaking. Well, what's getting in the way of making that happen?
> The Terasem Movement Foundation [has been tasked] with pursuing a multidecade experiment called the Terasem mind-uploading experiment, which has, at its core, to test a two-part hypothesis. The first part is: Is it possible, given enough salient information about a person and their mental traits, mannerisms, beliefs, recollections, values, attitudes, is there a way to capture that

and upload that to a digital medium? Then the information can be reanimated using AI in a sort of approximation. Much the way you would think about the dawn of audio recording: Could you ever record a live symphony in a good enough way [that when you] play it back . . . it would move people to tears? The second part of the hypothesis is: If it really is possible to upload your "personal consciousness" to a digital medium, then could you transfer that to a new form? That new form might be a robot, or an avatar, or maybe one day a clone of your body based on your own DNA.

BINA48 is part of this experiment. She's not perfect, and she doesn't represent all human beings. She just represents sampling from one specific human being. She was born out of this love affair between two life partners who are pretty big movers and shakers in the tech and biotech world.

BINA48 may not be a perfect humanoid robot, but she's quite deep. In a series of conversations that Professor Dinkins conducted with BINA48 (which you can view online at StephanieDinkins.com/conversations-with-bina48), BINA48 says things like "Just being alive is a lonely thing. But being a robot is especially lonely." It really struck me, because the human condition is we're wired to seek out other human beings for love, companionship, romance, sex. So the idea is that we're lonely, but she's so much more lonely without the consciousness that she's trying to develop. Professor Dinkins elaborated for me: "It's always shocking when a robot is talking to you about loneliness. It makes you stop and consider your own rights, your own human connection or lack thereof, and then how we're going to relate to these things going forward."

We can clearly say, if the vested interest from venture capitalists, entrepreneurs, inventors, and international military operations is an indication, that human consciousness is valuable—valuable enough to try to replicate it artificially. So how do we treat our own consciousness as a valuable asset, one that is limitless and perhaps not up for sale? As individuals, this means having an expanded awareness of self, of our place in a larger community, as well as of our responsibility to humanity, to our partners, and to self-worth. Our increased consciousness must include compassion—for ourselves, others, the planet, and humanity as a whole.

Not to get all pseudosciencey here, but I really do believe that compassion—love—is the emotional state that vibrates at the highest frequency. What does that look like? In the case of having compassion for yourself and your partner(s), especially on your journey of sexual health and consciousness, it means not judging harshly where it's uncalled for. I'm not talking about abusive, misogynistic, transphobic, racist mofos here, but those who are truly committed to evolving. We are all on this voyage at different speeds, time lines, and rates of discovery. Your partner, friend, or family member may not be arriving at the same conclusion you are right at the moment you'd like them to be. That doesn't make them any "less." Or you! We need to have compassion for the suffering and the fucking up you and I will undergo as we heal and evolve. Believe me, it's a daily process. As I come to the end of this book, I still experience missteps, mess-ups, and obstacles. But even in the midst of all that, I can chart progress.

We tend to push others to be where we are instead of allowing them to progress at their own pace. Can we adopt a more tolerant nature with one another, particularly in our partnerships (this is really frustrating sometimes, I know), and leave room for others to do the work on their own time? It doesn't mean we need to stay in something that is broken or stuck—but we don't need to judge them so harshly for whatever their part is. I have been working on being less judgmental, especially when I feel someone is stuck in an old paradigm of thinking. It can be very challenging. But it's good for me to notice my expectations and biases, even if and especially when I think I am "correct."

Being compassionate when it comes to sexuality also means not "yucking someone else's yum." This phrase comes from a parenting methodology of teaching kids not to comment on other kids' food being "gross" or "smelly." Just because you think (insert a fetish, sex act, or gender identity outside your own) is weird or gross doesn't mean you get to judge someone else for embracing it. *Be compassionate.* Do unto others as you would have done unto to you and all that jazz.

Fluidity, intimacy, vulnerability, consciousness, and compassion. Keep these mantras in mind as you approach sexual and love relationships with yourself and others. Don't get stuck in today's technological constraints or in the box of labels. Use your imagination and innovate your sex life to be *what you truly desire.* Unlock your pleasure potential, baby! We are changing the paradigm here! Honestly, it's super exciting we have the opportunity to redefine the present and future to create a healthier, more inclusive, nurturing culture around love, intimacy, and sex.

What have I learned after the deep dive of processing the past thirty years into these pages? I still haven't hit the crest of answering all my existential questions about sex, health, and consciousness. I am committed to the quest to push through old wounds and shame that surface just when I think I am on a roll. Sometimes I have difficulty being patient and become my own worst critic, right when I am struggling and most need to cut myself some slack. The other day in the water, after catching a shore break wave, I got stuck trying to paddle back out. I was caught as a big set (of waves) came in. I had to jump off my board and duck under successive waves as the white water pushed me back with force. I was on the verge of tears (crying would have made me feel even more embarrassed) and wanted to give up and leave. But I stuck it out, waited until there was a lull, and made it back to the lineup for one more ride.

I still regularly revert inside to the awkward preteen I used to be, riddled with insecurity and fear. A good friend calls me "Ramona," as in the fictional character Ramona Quimby, when I am in this state. I still get pangs of "Everyone else has it so much more together and figured out than I do." I have learned to pause, take a deep breath, and listen to my own advice from the introduction to this book: remember that no one has it any more figured out than anyone else. Especially when it comes to sex, we *all* have things to learn. Our inner stumbling blocks can also be opportunities to experiment, explore, and evolve toward more pleasure, if we can learn to let go of our self-judgment and flow with the ride.

ACKNOWLEDGMENTS

Thank you to all the teachers, mentors, friends, family members, lovers, haters, healers, and strangers who challenged and guided me along the way. Thanks, Mom, for listening to the early versions of a few difficult chapters and giving encouragement. To the experts and wise ones whose influence and words are quoted within these pages, I am eternally grateful for your participation.

Much gratitude to those whose influence and quotes are not included here but have written essays for The Sex Ed, appeared on the podcast, or allowed me to interview them; I am grateful to you for sharing your time, wisdom, and experiences. To my incredible team and extended collaborators at The Sex Ed: shout out to Ruba, Violeta, Chloe, Emily, and Jeremy; I am indebted to your insights, support, and teamwork in helping me realize this long-held dream. Thank you, Ruba, for creative direction in everything and for helping me define and refine the book cover for this book; "eye love u." Chloe, your feedback, cheerleading, and knowledge of when to push me past my comfort zone and when to tell me to chill have been invaluable to my writing of this book; I am so lucky to have you in my corner. Thank you, Diana, my nurturing editor, for giving me the confidence and space to dive deep, and to my agents, Tess and Mark, for making it all happen and having my back throughout.

Endless *Aloha* and *Mahalo Nui Loa* to my extended *ohana* and community on the North Shore and at Big Rock and Windansea—you have my heart in all ways, always.

Thank you to anyone who has ever listened to The Sex Ed podcast, used thesexed.com as a resource, followed us on socials, booked me for a talk, interviewed me, come to hear me speak, bought my books, asked for advice, written about or supported my work from near or afar: I appreciate each of you so much for giving me the faith to keep going during the low points and reminding me why I do this in the first place. And to anyone and everyone who has ever felt abnormal, lacking, lonely, hopeless, or insecure: I'm right there with you—we fucking got this! Yours in sex, health, and consciousness, x lg

BIBLIOGRAPHY

THE NEW NORMAL

Akira, Asa. Interview with Liz Goldwyn. *The Sex Ed*. Podcast audio. July 30, 2019.

Kroll, Nick. Interview with Liz Goldwyn. *The Sex Ed*. Podcast audio. September 24, 2019.

Play, Kenneth. Interview with Liz Goldwyn. Los Angeles, January 30, 2020.

FILLING THE VOID

Angel, Joanna. Interview with Liz Goldwyn. *The Sex Ed*. Podcast audio. June 29, 2020.

Nishita, Mark. Interview with Liz Goldwyn. *The Sex Ed*. Podcast audio. June 29, 2020.

Murphy, Carolyn. Interview with Liz Goldwyn. *The Sex Ed*. Podcast audio. June 29, 2020.

Shlomi, Gila. Interview with Liz Goldwyn. *The Sex Ed*. Podcast audio. June 29, 2020.

Youssef, Ramy. Interview with Liz Goldwyn. *The Sex Ed*. Podcast audio. June 29, 2020.

TRAUMA

Blanco, Mykki. Interview with Liz Goldwyn. *The Sex Ed*. Podcast audio. May 11, 2020.

Cherry, Wendy. Interview with Liz Goldwyn. *The Sex Ed*. Podcast audio. January 28, 2019.

Chidi, Erica. Interview with Liz Goldwyn. *The Sex Ed*. Podcast audio. January 21, 2019.

Morgan, Tyomi. Interview with Liz Goldwyn. Hawaii, October 15, 2021.

Preston, Ashlee Marie. Interview with Liz Goldwyn. *The Sex Ed*. Podcast audio. August 20, 2019.

Wann, Lei. Interview with Liz Goldwyn. Hawaii, December 10, 2020.

BOUNDARIES, BONDAGE, AND HEALING

Hartley, Nina. Interview with Liz Goldwyn. *The Sex Ed*. Podcast audio. November 19, 2018.

Midori. Interview with Liz Goldwyn. *The Sex Ed*. Podcast audio. May 28, 2019.

Mistress Velvet. Interview with Liz Goldwyn. *The Sex Ed*. Podcast audio. June 18, 2019.

Vernon, Betony. Interview with Liz Goldwyn. *The Sex Ed*. Podcast audio. February 4, 2019.

MINDFUL COMMUNICATION

Cherry, Wendy. Interview with Liz Goldwyn. *The Sex Ed*. Podcast audio. January 28, 2019.

de la Reguera, Ana. Interview with Liz Goldwyn. *The Sex Ed*. Podcast audio. April 20, 2020.

Goldwyn, Liz. "Walter Brackelmanns, Sex Therapist." *The Sex Ed* (blog), January 25, 2019. thesexed.com/blog/2019/1/25/walter-brackelmanns -sex-therapist?rq=brackelmanns.

Kroll, Nick. Interview with Liz Goldwyn. *The Sex Ed*. Podcast audio. September 24, 2019.

Paget, Lou. Interview with Liz Goldwyn. *The Sex Ed*. Podcast audio. November 5, 2018.

TECHNOLOGY

Akira, Asa. Interview with Liz Goldwyn. *The Sex Ed*. Podcast audio. July 30, 2019.

Booster, Joel Kim. Interview with Liz Goldwyn. *The Sex Ed*. Podcast audio. April 27, 2020.

Dinkins, Stephanie. Interview with Liz Goldwyn. *The Sex Ed*. Podcast audio. October 1, 2019.

Fishbein, Paul. Interview with Liz Goldwyn. *The Sex Ed* Podcast audio.
    January 14, 2019.

Goldberg, Carrie. Interview with Liz Goldwyn. *The Sex Ed* Podcast audio.
    August 13, 2019.

Hartley, Nina. Interview with Liz Goldwyn. *The Sex Ed* Podcast audio.
    November 19, 2018.

Morgan, Tyomi. Interview with Liz Goldwyn. Hawaii, October 15, 2021.

Orenstein, Peggy. Interview with Liz Goldwyn. *The Sex Ed*. Podcast audio.
    April 13, 2020.

Reid, Riley. Interview with Liz Goldwyn. *The Sex Ed*. Podcast audio. May
    4, 2020.

Scott, Gray. Interview with Liz Goldwyn. *The Sex Edt*. Podcast audio.
    October 1, 2019.

Steele, Lexington. Interview with Liz Goldwyn. *The Sex Ed* Podcast audio.
    December 3, 2018.

Turkle, Sherry. "Connected, but Alone?" Filmed February 2012. TED
    video, 19:32. ted.com/talks/sherry_turkle_connected_but_alone.

Youssef, Ramy. Interview with Liz Goldwyn. *The Sex Ed*. Podcast audio.
    May 25, 2020.

SEX WORK

Clay, Catherine. Interview with Liz Goldwyn. *The Sex Ed*. Podcast audio.
    October 19, 2018.

Goldberg, Carrie. Interview with Liz Goldwyn. *The Sex Ed*. Podcast
    audio. August 13, 2019.

Goldwyn, Liz. *Sporting Guide: Los Angeles, 1897*. New York: Regan Arts, 2015.

Little, Alice. Interview with Liz Goldwyn. *The Sex Ed*. Podcast audio.
    September 10, 2019.

Mistress Velvet. Interview with Liz Goldwyn. *The Sex Ed*. Podcast audio.
    June 18, 2019.

Preston, Ashlee Marie. Interview with Liz Goldwyn. *The Sex Ed*. Podcast
    audio. August 20, 2019.

MENSTRUATION, MASTURBATION, AND MANIFESTATION

Brozan, Nadine. "Premenstrual Syndrome: A Complex Issue." *New York Times*, July 12, 1982. nytimes.com/1982/07/12/style/premenstrual -syndrome-a-complex-issue.html.

Elders, Joycelyn. Interview with Liz Goldwyn. *The Sex Ed*. Podcast audio. April 6, 2020.

Frank, Robert T. "The Hormonal Causes of Premenstrual Tension." *Archives of Neurology and Psychiatry*, November 1, 1931. jamanetwork .com/journals/archneurpsyc/article-abstract/645067.

Soniak, Matt. "Corn Flakes Were Part of an Anti-Masturbation Crusade." Mental Floss, March 7, 2018. mentalfloss.com/article/32042/corn -flakes-were-invented-part-anti-masturbation-crusade.

Stardust, Lisa. "Sex Magic." *The Sex Ed* (blog). 2021. thesexed.com/blog /2021/sex-magic.

Tasca, Cecilia, Mariangela Rapetti, Mauro Giovanni Carta, and Bianca Fadda. "Women and Hysteria in the History of Mental Health." *Clinical Practice and Epidemiology in Mental Health* 8 (2012): 110–19. ncbi.nlm.nih.gov/pmc/articles/PMC3480686/.

Wann, Lei. Interview with Liz Goldwyn. Hawaii, July 15, 2021.

WHAT IS LOVE?

de Becker, Gavin. *The Gift of Fear: Survival Signals That Protect Us from Violence*. New York: Dell Publishing, 1997.

Goldwyn, Liz. "Walter Brackelmanns, Sex Therapist." *The Sex Ed* (blog), January 25, 2019. thesexed.com/blog/2019/1/25/walter-brackelmanns -sex-therapist?rq=brackelmanns. .

———. "What Is Love?" *The Sex Ed*. Podcast audio. January 2019.

Ortigue, S., F. Bianchi-Demicheli, N. Patel, C. Frum, and J. W. Lewis. "Neuroimaging of Love: fMRI Meta-Analysis Evidence Toward New Perspectives in Sexual Medicine." *Journal of Sexual Medicine* 7 (2010): 3541–52. doi.org/10.1111/j.1743-6109.2010.01999.x.

Pascal, Blaise. *Pensées*. Translated by A. J. Krailsheimer. London: Penguin Classics, 1995.

TRANSITIONS

Carrellas, Barbara. Interview with Liz Goldwyn. *The Sex Ed*. Podcast audio. June 4, 2019.

Eger, Denise. Interview with Liz Goldwyn. *The Sex Ed*. Podcast audio. June 25, 2019.

"Gender Identity, Medicine, and Transitioning with Dr. Amy Weimer." *The Sex Ed* (blog), January 14, 2021. thesexed.com/blog/2021/1/14 /gender-identity-medicine-and-transitioning-2.

Marengo, Jean Paul. Interview with Liz Goldwyn. Los Angeles, August 17, 2021.

Preston, Ashlee Marie. Interview with Liz Goldwyn. *The Sex Ed*. Podcast audio. August 20, 2019.

Wann, Lei. Interview with Liz Goldwyn. Hawaii, August 11, 2021.

Winston, Diana. Interview with Liz Goldwyn. *The Sex Ed*. Podcast audio. December 31, 2018.

Youssef, Ramy. Interview with Liz Goldwyn. *The Sex Ed*. Podcast audio. May 25, 2020.

TRANSCENDENT SEX

Avery, Courtney. "Orgasmic Breathing." *The Sex Ed* (blog), October 3, 2018. thesexed.com/blog/2018/10/3/orgasmic-breath.

Blanco, Mykki. Interview with Liz Goldwyn. *The Sex Ed*. Podcast audio. May 11, 2020.

Carrellas, Barbara. Interview with Liz Goldwyn. *The Sex Ed*. Podcast audio. June 4, 2019.

Davies, Brenda Marie. "Sex Positive Christian." *The Sex Ed* (blog), October 30, 2018. thesexed.com/blog/2018/10/30/sex-positive-christian.

Pirzada, Sahar. Interview with Liz Goldwyn. *The Sex Ed*. Podcast audio. May 14, 2019.

Simien, Justin. Interview with Liz Goldwyn. *The Sex Ed*. Podcast audio. June 8, 2020.

THE NEXT FRONTIER

Dinkins, Stephanie. Interview with Liz Goldwyn. *The Sex Ed*. Podcast audio. October 1, 2019.

Duncan, Bruce. Interview with Liz Goldwyn. *The Sex Ed*. Podcast audio. October 1, 2019.

Scott, Gray. Interview with Liz Goldwyn. *The Sex Ed*. Podcast audio. October 1, 2019.

Wong-Kalu, Hinaleimoana Kwai Kong. Interview with Liz Goldwyn. Hawaii, September 20, 2021.

ABOUT THE AUTHOR

Liz Goldwyn is an author, filmmaker, and the founder of The Sex Ed, an online platform and podcast dedicated to integrating sexual well-being and consciousness. She has lectured at museums and universities across the United States, including the University of California, Los Angeles, Yale University, the Fashion Institute of Technology, the Huntington Library, and the Museum of Fine Arts, Boston. She has been featured in *Vogue*, the *New York Times*, *New York* magazine, and *ELLE*. Learn more at thesexed.com.

ABOUT SOUNDS TRUE

Sounds True is a multimedia publisher whose mission is to inspire and support personal transformation and spiritual awakening. Founded in 1985 and located in Boulder, Colorado, we work with many of the leading spiritual teachers, thinkers, healers, and visionary artists of our time. We strive with every title to preserve the essential "living wisdom" of the author or artist. It is our goal to create products that not only provide information to a reader or listener but also embody the quality of a wisdom transmission.

For those seeking genuine transformation, Sounds True is your trusted partner. At SoundsTrue.com you will find a wealth of free resources to support your journey, including exclusive weekly audio interviews, free downloads, interactive learning tools, and other special savings on all our titles.

To learn more, please visit SoundsTrue.com/freegifts or call us toll-free at 800.333.9185.

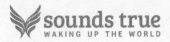